Gastrointestinal Issues and Complications

Editors

DEBORAH WEATHERSPOON
DEBRA HENLINE SULLIVAN

CRITICAL CARE NURSING CLINICS OF NORTH AMERICA

www.ccnursing.theclinics.com

Consulting Editor
JAN FOSTER

March 2018 • Volume 30 • Number 1

ELSEVIER

1600 John F. Kennedy Boulevard • Suite 1800 • Philadelphia, Pennsylvania, 19103-2899

http://www.theclinics.com

CRITICAL CARE NURSING CLINICS OF NORTH AMERICA Volume 30, Number 1
March 2018 ISSN 0899-5885, ISBN-13: 978-0-323-58150-9

Editor: Kerry Holland
Developmental Editor: Laura Fisher

Critical Care Nursing Clinics of North America (ISSN 0899-5885) is published quarterly by Elsevier Inc., 360 Park Avenue South, New York, NY 10010-1710. Months of issue are March, June, September, and December. Business and Editorial Offices: 1600 John F. Kennedy Blvd., Suite 1800, Philadelphia, PA 19103-2899. Periodicals postage paid at New York, NY and additional mailing offices. Subscription prices are $155.00 per year for US individuals, $385.00 per year for US institutions, $100.00 per year for US students and residents, $200.00 per year for Canadian individuals, $483.00 per year for Canadian institutions, $230.00 per year for international individuals, $483.00 per year for international institutions and $115.00 per year for Canadian and international students/residents. To receive student/resident rate, orders must be accompanied by name of affiliated institution, data of term, and the *signature* of program/residency coordinator on institution letterhead. Orders will be billed at individual rate until proof of status is received. Foreign air speed delivery is included in all *Clinics* subscription prices. All prices are subject to change without notice. **POSTMASTER:** Send address changes to *Critical Care Nursing Clinics of North America*, Elsevier Health Sciences Division, Subscription Customer Service, 3251 Riverport Lane, Maryland Heights, MO 63043. **Customer Service: 1-800-654-2452 (US and Canada); 314-447-8871 (outside US and Canada). Fax: 314-447-8029. E-mail:** JournalsCustomerService-usa@elsevier.com **(for print support) and** JournalsOnlineSupport-usa@elsevier.com **(for online support).**

Reprints. For copies of 100 or more of articles in this publication, please contact the Commercial Reprints Department, Elsevier Inc., 360 Park Avenue South, New York, New York, 10010-1710; Tel.: 212-633-3874, Fax: 212-633-3820, and E-mail: reprints@elsevier.com.

Critical Care Nursing Clinics of North America is covered in *MEDLINE/PubMed (Index Medicus), International Nursing Index, Nursing Citation Index, Cumulative Index to Nursing and Allied Health Literature,* and *RNdex Top 100.*

Contributors

CONSULTING EDITOR

JAN FOSTER, PhD, APRN, CNS
Formerly, Associate Professor, College of Nursing, Texas Woman's University, Houston, Texas; Currently, President, Nursing Inquiry and Intervention, Inc, The Woodlands, Texas

EDITORS

DEBORAH WEATHERSPOON, PhD, MSN, RN, CRNA, COI
Faculty, MSN Leadership and Management Program, College of Health Science, School of Nursing, Walden University, Minneapolis, Minnesota

DEBRA HENLINE SULLIVAN, PhD, MSN, RN, CNE, COI
Faculty, Core MSN Program, College of Health Science, School of Nursing, Walden University, Minneapolis, Minnesota

AUTHORS

MARY BEMKER, PhD, PsyS, LADC, LPCC, CCFP, CNE, RN
Contributing Faculty, College of Health Sciences, School of Nursing, Walden University, Minneapolis, Minnesota

LORETTA BOND, RN, PhD, CNE
Assistant Professor of Nursing, Gordon E. Inman College of Health Sciences & Nursing, Belmont University, Nashville, Tennessee

ANGELA COLLINS-YODER, PhD, RN, CCNS, ACNS BC
Clinical Professor, Capstone College of Nursing, The University of Alabama, Tuscaloosa, Alabama; Critical Care Clinical Specialist, Ascension Sacred Heart Health System, Pensacola, Florida

CATHY A. COOPER, EdD, MSN, RN, CNE
Associate Professor, School of Nursing, Middle Tennessee State University, Murfreesboro, Tennessee

MICHELE DUNSTAN, MSN, RN, CCRN
Pediatric Trauma Coordinator, Lehigh Valley Health Network, Allentown, Pennsylvania

DEBORAH L. ELLISON, PhD, MSN, BSN
Professor, School of Nursing, Austin Peay State University, Clarksville, Tennessee

FRANCISCA CISNEROS FARRAR, EdD, MSN, RN
Professor, School of Nursing, Austin Peay State University, Clarksville, Tennessee

TERESA D. FERGUSON, DNP, RN, CNE
Associate Professor, Department of Nursing, Morehead State University, 201M Center for Health, Education and Research, Staff Nurse, Woman's Care Unit, St. Claire HealthCare, Morehead, Kentucky

CHRISTINE FRAZER, PhD, CNS, CNE, RN
MSN Senior Core Faculty, College of Health Sciences, School of Nursing, Walden University, Minneapolis, Minnesota

VINCENT P. HALL, PhD, RN, CNE
MSN Program Director, School of Nursing, Walden University, Minneapolis, Minnesota

BETH HALLMARK, RN, PhD, CHSE
Assistant Professor of Nursing, Gordon E. Inman College of Health Sciences & Nursing, Belmont University, Nashville, Tennessee

STACIA M. HAYS, DNP, CPNP-PC, CCTC, CNE
Clinical Assistant Professor, College of Nursing University of Florida, Gainesville, Florida

LESLIE HUSSEY, PhD, CNE, RN
Nursing PhD Program Coordinator, College of Health Sciences, School of Nursing, Walden University, Minneapolis, Minnesota

ROBIN M. LAWSON, DNP
Senior Associate Dean, Academic Programs, The University of Alabama, Capstone College of Nursing, Tuscaloosa, Alabama

MELANIE McGHEE, MSN, RN, ACNP-BC
Structural Heart Nurse Practitioner, Department of Structural Heart, Saint Thomas West Hospital, Nashville, Tennessee

CHERYL W. McGINNIS, DNP, ARNP-BC, CCTC
DNP Program Coordinator, College of Health Sciences, School of Nursing, Walden University, Minneapolis, Minnesota

SHELLEY C. MOORE, PhD, MSN, RN
Associate Professor, School of Nursing, Middle Tennessee State University, Murfreesboro, Tennessee

SUZANNE S. PUENTES, BSN, RN, CCRN
Patient Care Specialist, Children's Emergency Room, Lehigh Valley Health Network, Allentown, Pennsylvania

MARCIA A. PUGH, DNP, RN, MBA, HCM, MSN
Grants, Research and Outreach of West AL Division, Tombigbee Healthcare Authority, Demopolis, Alabama

MARIA A. REVELL, PhD, RN, MSN, COI
Associate Professor, School of Nursing, Tennessee State University, Nashville, Tennessee

ROBIN SQUELLATI, PhD, APRN-C
Core Faculty, MSN SP Program, Walden University, Sparks, Nevada

PATTI P. URSO, PhD, APRN, ANP-BC, FNP, CNE
Faculty and Specialization Coordinator, Nursing Education, School of Nursing, Walden University, Minneapolis, Minnesota

TERESA D. WELCH, EdD, RN, NEA-BC
Assistant Professor, Capstone College of Nursing, The University of Alabama, Tuscaloosa, Alabama

Contents

Proper functioning within the gastrointestinal (GI) system is essential to immune integrity. Autoimmune diseases (ADs) can disrupt GI integrity and cause serious derangements of organ function. ADs exist on a continuum of mild to severe. Life-threatening presentations of ADs can lead to rapid clinical demise. In addition, the medications used to control ADs can precipitate gastric bleeding and predispose patients to sepsis in critical care. AD treatment focuses on diminishing symptoms through reducing autoantibody production that leads to cytokine release. This article details common and rare presentations of acute ADs associated with GI manifestations in critically ill patients.

Critically ill patients have increased metabolic requirements and must rely on the administration of nutritional therapy to meet those demands. Yet, according to research almost half of all hospitalized patients are not fed, are underfed, or are malnourished while in the hospital. This article demonstrates the importance of early feedings in critical care unit and the available options open to nurses supporting initiation and management of early feedings. Enteral nutrition has proven to be an important therapeutic strategy for improving the outcomes of critically ill patients, and the critical care nurse plays an integral role in their success.

Mesenteric ischemia is an uncommon disease most often seen in the elderly. This disease results from blood flow in the mesenteric circulation that inadequately meets metabolic needs of the visceral organs and, if untreated, eventually leads to necrosis of the bowel wall. Mesenteric ischemia is divided into 2 types: acute mesenteric ischemia (AMI) and chronic mesenteric ischemia (CMI). Delayed diagnosis of CMI can lead to AMI. AMI is associated with extremely high mortalities. Early diagnosis via computed tomography angiography and prompt revascularization via endovascular therapy are recommended for symptomatic patients who have not developed bowel ischemia and necrosis.

indicated when failure to gain weight, irritability, swallowing difficulties, regurgitation, and respiratory complications occur and should trigger referral to pediatric specialists. This article shares information about uncomplicated GER, GERD, and symptoms of these diagnoses, common screening tests, and treatment options.

CRITICAL CARE NURSING CLINICS OF NORTH AMERICA

ISSUE OF RELATED INTEREST

Nursing Clinics, June 2017 (Vol. 52, Issue 2)
Fluids and Electrolytes
Joshua Squires, *Editor*
Available at: http://nursing.theclinics.com

THE CLINICS ARE AVAILABLE ONLINE!
Access your subscription at:
www.theclinics.com

Preface

Gastrointestinal Issues and Complications

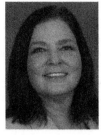
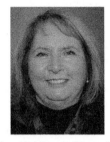

Deborah Weatherspoon,
PhD, MSN, RN, CRNA, COI

Debra Henline Sullivan, PhD,
MSN, RN, CNE, COI

Editors

Gastrointestinal (GI) dysfunction and failure are common problems in the critically ill patient, as a primary reason for admission or developing as part of multiple organ dysfunction syndrome. Delayed gastric emptying, abnormal motility patterns, and impaired intestinal barrier integrity are commonly observed in the critical care unit and are associated with complications and morbidities that may affect survival. In this issue of *Critical Care Nursing Clinics of North America*, a wide variety of primary and secondary causes of GI dysfunction are discussed.

Complications related to inflammation and infection, either as a primary or as a secondary outcome, cause serious morbidity in both adults and pediatric populations. The epidemic proportion of *Clostridium difficile* infection gives cause for concern, especially for vulnerable populations as adults over age 65; further *C difficile* infection is described by the Centers for Disease Control and Prevention as an urgent threat that is very difficult to manage in any population and more so in patients with critical illness. Moore reviews clinical manifestations of the infection, outlines both medical and surgical treatment options, and discusses risk factors, diagnostics, and ways to improve prevention strategies. Squellati reviews the role of antibiotics leading to *C difficile* infection and reviews the pros and cons of probiotics as a potential treatment. Yet another pathogenic GI infection is shiga toxin–producing *E coli*. While this is a significant threat to all age groups, it is especially dangerous for young children, who are prone to develop a more severe illness, hemolytic uremic syndrome (HUS). Puentes and Dunstan focus on the pediatric population and the potentially life-threatening complication of HUS. In their review, a summary of pathogenesis, clinical presentation, diagnosis, and symptom management is discussed.

Crit Care Nurs Clin N Am 30 (2018) xiii–xv
https://doi.org/10.1016/j.cnc.2017.10.016
0899-5885/18/© 2017 Published by Elsevier Inc.

ccnursing.theclinics.com

Ellison provides insight into the diagnosis, treatment, and management of acute diverticulitis and potential complication and provides a case study that is interesting and informative. Cooper and Urso review the signs and symptoms of gastroesophageal reflux and provide the latest evidence-based practice for the treatment and care in the adult population. Ferguson brings information regarding reflux and regurgitation in the infant population.

Revell, Pugh, and McGhee review traumatic injuries that directly or indirectly lead to bowel injuries and include management of hemodynamic unstable patients and its effect on the bowel. GI bleeding in both the upper and lower GI system is a frequent problem seen in critical care patients. Farrar reviews various disorders leading to GI bleeds and treatment options. Lawson reports specifically on complications associated with decreased circulation to the GI system and mesenteric ischemia.

Conditions that affect the immune system and the medications used to treat autoimmune disease can disrupt GI integrity. Collins-Yoder looks at autoimmune diseases and the medications often prescribed and potential GI complications. Hall focuses on HIV patients who are on antiviral medication as well as those living with AIDS who present with GI complications. Updated information is presented for both these patient populations.

The critical care nurse has excellent assessment and monitoring skills; however, GI issues can be more complex, often presenting with vague yet serious issues. This issue includes three articles related to assessment and management of GI issues. Bond and Hallmark discuss nursing education, or skills training, in a simulated setting using an algorithm that incorporates the Sequential Organ Failure Tool and the Gastrointestinal Failure Tool. According to recent research, almost half of all hospitalized patients are not fed, are underfed, or are malnourished while in the hospital due to increased metabolic needs while hospitalized. Welch addresses the importance of early feedings while in critical care, and the available options, including enteral and parenteral feedings, that support initiation and management of early feedings. Frazer, Hussey, and Bemker discuss the critical care patient at risk of GI complications due to motility disorders. These patients require close monitoring and an acute awareness of the causation, symptoms, and treatment of various GI motility disorders, including gastroparesis, ileus, and toxic megacolon. Another group requiring specialized critical care is patients experiencing end-stage liver failure or those preparing for a liver transplant. McGinnis and Hays describe the vital role nurses play caring this population prior to, and immediately after, transplantation.

We hope that this update on GI complications increases awareness of the potential problems, either as a primary concern or as a comorbid one, in the critical care patient. The authors for each article have provided an updated review of literature and presented the current evidence-based care evidence to inform nursing practice for the critical care population.

Deborah Weatherspoon, PhD, MSN, RN, CRNA, COI
College of Health Science
School of Nursing MSN Leadership and Management Program
Walden University
100 Washington Avenue South, Suite 900
Minneapolis, MN 55401, USA

Debra Henline Sullivan, PhD, MSN, RN, CNE, COI
College of Health Science
School of Nursing Core MSN Program
Walden University
100 Washington Avenue South, Suite 900
Minneapolis, MN 55401, USA

E-mail addresses:
Deborah.Weatherspoon@waldenu.edu (D. Weatherspoon)
Debra.Sullivan@waldenu.edu (D.H. Sullivan)

Gastrointestinal Manifestations of Autoimmune Diseases Requiring Critical Care

Angela Collins-Yoder, PhD, RN, CCNS, ACNS BC[a,b,*]

KEYWORDS

- Autoimmune hepatitis • Autoimmune pancreatitis
- Catastrophic antiphospholipid syndrome • Systemic lupus erythematosus
- Immunosuppressive medications • Biological medications
- Disease-modifying medications

KEY POINTS

- Gastrointestinal organs have specific autoimmune diseases that can present to critical care, primarily the liver, pancreas, and intestines.
- There are systemic autoimmune diseases that present with gastrointestinal manifestations.
- Most interventions for autoimmune diseases are linked to immune pharmacology and decreasing circulating antibodies.
- Autoimmune diseases are often clinical diagnoses and require extensive laboratory testing.

INTRODUCTION

Gastrointestinal (GI) integrity, appropriate liver function, and beneficial bacterial flora are vital to overall immune system competence.[1] It is, therefore, not surprising that both autoimmune diseases (ADs) expressed within the GI tract and systemic ADs can acutely present signs and symptoms within the GI system. There are estimated to be 50 million persons in the United States with ADs.[2] Women predominate the statistics reported for each of the 80 to 100 AD spectra. This sex-associated incidence is attributed to multiple theories. One theme that is repeated through each theory is the high reactivity of the female immune system to circulating self-antigens. Additionally, AD often presents as 2 or more overlapping autoimmune processes within a single patient.[2] AD diseases are chronic and exist on a continuum of mild to severe. The intent

The author has no financial disclosures and does not speak for any of the pharmacology that is included in the article.
[a] Capstone College of Nursing, The University of Alabama, Box 870358, Tuscaloosa, AL 35487, USA; [b] Sacred Heart of Pensacola, Pensacola, FL, USA
* 8370 Foxtail Loop, Pensacola, FL 32526.
E-mail address: acollins-yoder@ua.edu

of this article is to review the acute clinical presentations of each GI-associated AD and to focus on high acuity interventions. These interventions are primarily medical and grouped as antiinflammatory drugs, immunosuppression, disease-modifying medications, and biological pharmacology categories. The desired outcome of medication intervention is to decrease autoantibody formation and suppress subsequent generation of inflammatory cytokines. When caring for patients with ADs, the health care provider must focus on the correct diagnosis, correct drug, appropriate dose, and for a sufficient duration.

Three categories of GI patients require critical care for AD. These categories are organ-specific ADs, such as liver, pancreas, and intestinal. Next, there are clinical presentations of immune dysregulation, such as angioedema (AE) of the intestines leading to an acute abdomen. Finally, there are clinical presentations of systemic ADs that initially manifest with severe GI signs and symptoms. AD statistics in critical care populations describe that the frequent ADs requiring critical care were antiphospholipid syndrome (APS), systemic lupus erythematous (SLE), and rheumatoid arthritis (RA). Each of these AD types can have GI system manifestations. The mortality for patients with ADs in the critical care area ranged from 17% to 55% and was associated with high Acute Physiology and Chronic Health Evaluation scores.[3] Lungs are typically the first organ to fail in patients with ADs in critical care. Lung damage is attributed to the microcirculation damage from activated circulating cytokines.[3]

Gastrointestinal Autoimmune Diseases: Liver, Pancreas, Inflammatory Bowel Disease

Liver and normal immune function

Examining the immune role of the liver in the immune system reveals some unique aspects. The liver is more tolerant to antigens and also serves as the body's sentinel to preventing bacterial systemic spread. The highly vascularized liver is bombarded with blood-borne pathogens and antigenic substances from digestion. This workload of pathogen containment and antigen recognition is specific to the liver network of cells called antigen-presenting cells (APCs).[4] APC cells types include Kupffer cells, dendrite cells, and liver sinusoid epithelium cells. These APC cells defend the body from pathogens. Paradoxically, APCs also have the property of making the liver less immunologically reactive to antigens through T-cell suppression. In autoimmune hepatitis, for example, there is abnormal feedback or dysfunction in the APCs and T cells activate. T-cell activation leads to a production of a cascade of immune cytokines leading to hepatic cell destruction (**Fig. 1**, **Table 1**). The APC system is the reason that immunosuppressive medications can selectively be reduced after a liver transplant.[5]

Liver and autoimmune diseases

The 3 types of liver ADs are autoimmune hepatitis (AIH), primary biliary cirrhosis (PBC), and primary sclerosing cholangitis (PSC). Systemic immunoglobulin G4 (IgG4) disorder can also target the liver. AIH is a rare disease produced by the interaction between the environment and genetic vulnerability. The incidence of AIH is estimated to be about 1 per 200,000 cases in the United States, with most being women.[6] Twenty-five percent of AIH can present as acute liver failure to the critical care unit. Acute liver failure is typically recognized as a decreased level of consciousness, elevated liver enzymes, respiratory failure, and metabolic acidosis. Acute AIH is often refractory to the effects of steroids.

Severe AIH is a clinical diagnosis. Supporting patterns of findings are liver-biopsy-identified centrilobular zone 3 necrosis, autoantibodies, and hypergammaglobulinemia. AIH must be differentiated from acute viral hepatitis and drug-induced liver injury (DILI) through a scoring system of probability and tissue biopsy findings.[7] Treatment

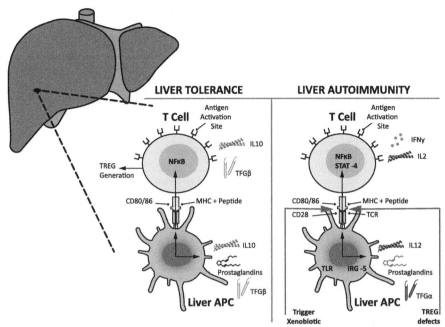

Fig. 1. Liver tolerance and pathogen clearance is regulated by the APC cells through chemical mediation between the APC and T cell. Note the cellular crosstalk between the multiple cytokines of the immune system between the APCs and T cells result in T-cell suppression. Liver autoimmune dysregulation is theorized to occur because of an interaction between genetics and T-cell (TREG) defect. The cellular chemical interactions lead to the production and release of cytokines that promote inflammation (see **Table 1** for the abbreviations used in the figure). (*Reproduced from* Grant CR, Liberal R. Liver immunology: how to reconcile tolerance with autoimmunity. Clin Res Hepatol Gastroenterol 2017;41(1):8. Copyright © 2017. Elsevier Masson SAS. All rights reserved.)

focuses on supportive therapy and pharmacologic immunosuppression[8] (**Table 2.**) Transplant evaluation also takes into consideration the likelihood of persistent autoimmune antibodies impacting the transplanted organ.[9]

PBC and PSC may also display overlapping disease presentations in acute AIH. Having both AIH and a concurrent cirrhosis or bile-obstructing disease makes an accurate diagnosis more complicated.[10] However, PBC and PSC are typically chronic conditions that most commonly appear in women in the fifth and sixth decade of life and are often known before an acute hospitalization. PBC and PSC may also be confounding concurrent diseases for patients with ADs admitted to critical care for other serious illnesses, such as sepsis.[6]

Recently a new subtype of IgG4 disorders has been linked to AIH. In this AIH clinical presentation, there are multiple thrombi of the liver tissues and destruction of the biliary process through fibrous. Serum elevation of immunoglobulin and lymph node enlargement are additional clinical findings. There are no specific diagnostic markers or evidence-based primary and chronic regimens for the care of these patients[10,11]

Autoimmune pancreas

There are 2 types of the autoimmune pancreas. In an acute presentation, the triggering event is typically pancreatic obstruction due to swelling and overwhelming abdominal

Table 1
Abbreviations used in Fig. 1

Acronyms	Terminology	Definition
IL-10	Interleukin 10	Cytokine that inhibits proinflammatory chemical release and has antiinflammatory properties
TGFβ	Transforming growth factor B	Cytokine controlling cell growth, cell proliferation, and apoptosis
Prostaglandins	Lipid compounds	Cytokine with cellular hormonal effects
MHC	Major histocompatibility protein	Proteins on surface of cells that helps immune system recognize antigens
TREG	Suppressor T cell	T cells that modulate tolerance to self-antigens
CD80/86	Cluster of differentiation 80/86	Proteins to initiate and maintain T-cell proliferation
IFNy	Interferon regulatory	Interferon factor regulatory factor 5 linked to destruction of self-tolerance leading to autoreactive B and T cells
TGFα	Transforming growth factor alpha	Cell signaling cytokine involved in systemic inflammation
TLR	Toll-like receptor	Transmembrane protein that recognizes antigens as a part of innate immunity
CD28	Cluster of differentiation 28	Protein expressed on T cell that is vital to T-cell survival
IL12	Interleukin 12	Cytokine produced during antigenic stimulation
IL2	Interleukin 2	Cytokine produced that regulates white blood cells
NFkB	Nuclear factor kappa light chain	Protein that is necessary to DNA transcription, cytokine production, and cell survival
STAT-4 gene	Signal transducer and activator transcription gene	Regulates the differentiation of T-helper cells
TCR	T-cell receptor site	Integral membrane proteins that activate T cells
IRG-5	Interferon subtype–immunity-related guanosine triphosphates	Activated cytokine that assists in clearance of pathogens

Data from Grant CR, Liberal R. Liver immunology: how to reconcile tolerance with autoimmunity. Clin Res Hepatol Gastroenterol 2017;41(1):6–16; and Gonzalez HC, Jafri S, Gordon SC. Management of acute hepatotoxicity including medical agents and liver support systems. Clin Liver Dis 2017;21(1):163–80.

pain. Acute pancreatitis is often associated with alcohol use, but this is an atypical finding with AD-associated pancreatitis. Autoimmune pancreatitis (AIP) type I is an organ-specific manifestation of a systemic IgG4 disorder. This immunologic disorder may impact any exocrine gland, such as the lacrimal, salivary, and parotid glands. IgG4 disorders exhibit a diverse set of clinical findings. In AIP type I presentations include tumorlike swelling of affected organs, infiltrate within the pancreas of IgG4-positive plasma cells, serum elevation in IgG4, and fibrosis that may result in obstruction.[12] AIP type II is also an autoimmune disease but differs within clinical findings and is not an IgG4-related disease. There is no immunoglobulin serum level elevation and often concurrently presents with patients with ulcerative colitis(UC).[13] AIP was first recognized in Japan but has a worldwide incidence. AIP must be differentiated from pancreatic cancer preventing unnecessary exploratory and Whipple surgical procedures. Both types of AIP are treated with immunosuppressive medications, typically steroids, remembering that type I AIP is characterized by relapsing episodes. The diagnosis of AIP is from computed tomography (CT) imaging and biopsy. Pharmacologic options for treatment are listed in **Table 2**.[14]

Inflammatory bowel diseases: ulcerative colitis and Crohn disease

UC and Crohn Disease (CD) are ADs that are commonly grouped together as inflammatory bowel diseases in the literature. UC is a chronic AD that has a genetic component and is typically controlled by immunosuppressive medications and diet. CD is characterized as intestinal inflammation and ulceration throughout the intestines and episodes of weight loss and food intolerance. CD may also have a genetic component. Both diseases start in adolescence or young adulthood. Patients with ADs with inflammatory bowel disease who require critical care can be admitted for any cause, such as a cardiovascular event.[15] However, patients with UC and patients with CD are particularly susceptible to experiencing a sepsis episode, triggered by a colon or intestinal perforation. Treatments to control the symptoms of these diseases may lead to renal insufficiency due to the dose of the immunosuppression medication. Other complications of these diseases, such as intra-abdominal abscesses and extensive immunosuppression, may also initiate a sepsis event. The focus of critical care admission and intervention is to assess the integrity of the immune system and to evaluate if the immunosuppression medications need adjustment or tapering to compliment recovery from the comorbid condition. This care calls for a collaborative effort between the interdisciplinary team of patient/family, nurse, intensivist, pharmacist, and rheumatologist.

Table 2
Drugs for autoimmune diseases of liver and pancreas

AD	Drug/Dose	Duration
PBC	UDCA 13–15 mg/kg/d Fibrates optimal dose unknown	Monitor for therapeutic response and follow liver enzymes
AIH	Steroids intravenous dosing during acute episodes Dosing recommendations varied Second-line medications Budesonide Azathioprine	Monitor for therapeutic response and monitor liver enzymes, kidney function, GI ulceration, osteonecrosis, osteoporosis, bleeding in urine and skin, excessive weight gain, bone marrow suppression
AIP	Steroids 0.6–1.0 mg/kg For 3–4 wk Second-line medications Rituximab Azathioprine 6-Mercaptopurine Mycophenolate	Monitor for therapeutic response and monitor liver enzymes, kidney function, GI ulceration, osteonecrosis, osteoporosis, bleeding in urine and skin, excessive weight gain, bone marrow suppression

Abbreviations: AIP, autoimmune pancreatitis; UDCA, ursodeoxycholic acid.
Data from Vallerand AH, Sanoski CA. Davis drug guide. 15th edition. Philadelphia: F.A. Davis; 2017.

Angioedema of abdominal organs an acute abdomen

AE is a bradykinin (BK)-mediated immune response that produces subcutaneous swelling of the dermis and tissues. This type of extravasation of fluid into the interstitial compartment is typically expressed in the upper airway but can also present as an acute abdomen. Clinical symptoms result because of an accumulation of vasoactive elements, particularly BK, histamine, and complement. AE may be drug induced, genetic, or idiopathic.[16] An acute abdomen is always a diagnostic challenge.[16] When AE of the abdomen is recognized, it is typically in patients with hereditary AE who have health care providers who are aware of the systemic effects of BK on the patients' tissues. AE of the abdomen appears as generalized swelling of all abdominal organs in the abdominal compartment on CT. Linking generalized abdominal swelling to the patients' history of angiotensin-converting enzyme inhibitor medications, exposure to a known allergen, or a history of hereditary AE is the key to making this diagnosis.[17] Because AE is a rare disease, unnecessary exploratory surgeries are often performed. Reports of these surgeries state that clinicians and radiologists rarely encounter the abdominal AE, and the radiological findings may be unclear.[18] Abdominal AE is rarely recognized outside of large academic centers. The pharmacology specific to treat the AE are within **Table 3** and because of cost are not often stocked in acute care pharmacies.

Systemic Autoimmune Diseases with Gastrointestinal Presentations: Antiphospholipid Syndrome, Systemic Lupus Erythematous, and Rheumatoid Arthritis

Antiphospholipid syndrome

The GI tract is highly vascular and rich in a network of capillary beds. This capillary concentration makes these organs vulnerable to AD processes within the vascular bed. The most obvious example is APS. APS may be a comorbidity with patients with systemic lupus or an isolated AD finding.[19] There are antibodies produced that have an exponential impact, each having a procoagulant effect. The end outcome of the release of these antibodies is both arterial and venous thrombosis with secondary placenta damage leading to fetal demise (**Table 4**). Giannakopoulos and Krilis[17] described APS as a 2-pronged hit resulting in thrombus that leads to organ failure.[17] In the first hit, the endothelium protective responses diminish; in the second, the coagulation cascades activate. The liver is especially vulnerable to APS with cases of hepatic infarction and portal hypertension as described in the literature. APS can also be linked to cases of intestinal angina and small bowel infarction.[20] APS can present to critical care as catastrophic APS (CAPS) with a rapid course of microthrombi release

Table 3 Angioedema medications		
Medication	**Classification**	**Mechanism of Action**
Human C1 inhibitor (Cinryze)	Proteinase inhibitors	Decrease release of BK (human blood derived)
Icatibant acetate (Firazyr)	BK B2 receptor antagonist	Decrease cytokine release, particularly BK
Ecallantide (Kalbitor)	Human kallikrein inhibitor	Selectively inhibits kallikrein thereby decreasing BK production

Data from Vallerand AH, Sanoski CA. Davis drug guide. 15th edition. Philadelphia: F.A. Davis; 2017; and Collins-Yoder AS. Angioedema: clinical presentations and pharmacological management. Dimens Crit Care Nurs 2016;35(4):181–9.

Table 4
Antiphospholipid antibodies: multiple sites of impact on coagulation and immunoregulatory mechanisms

Site of Antibodies Impact in APS	Outcome
Lipid peroxidative byproducts are increased	Procoagulant
Monocytes increase oxygen free radicals' production	Procoagulant
Disruption of annexin A5 shield (protein that inhibits coagulation)	Procoagulant
Impaired endothelial nitric oxide process that inhibits vascular relaxation	Vessel constriction
Platelet activation via apolipoprotein E receptor 2	Procoagulant
B-cell activating factor	Procoagulant
Antibody-mediated activation of complement C3 and C5	Fetal loss

Data from Giannakopoulos B, Krilis SA. The pathogenesis of the antiphospholipid syndrome. N Engl J Med 2013;368(11):1033–44.

and T-producing organ failure.[21] Typically, the liver, lungs, and kidneys are the first organs to fail because of each organ's extensive capillary beds. The cornerstones of CAPS treatment are to administer intravenous anticoagulants, immunosuppressive agents, and plasma apheresis to decrease circulating antibody volume.

Systemic lupus erythematous
SLE is an AD in which there are autoantibodies to the nuclear matter of patients' own cells. It is a complex disease with heterogeneous findings. SLE can be triggered by drug ingestion and is one of the only ADs that is more aggressive in pregnancy. This antibody release can affect all cellular components of the body, including the GI system.[20] A retrospective database review in Britain found in their patient cohort that 50% of the patients with SLE had abdominal complaints.[21] The larger percentage of complaints were found to be mild and linked to the medication's side effects. There were rare reports of acute illness with SLE. The acuity was increased when both SLE and APS were present. Acute presentations of intestinal angina, AIH, API, and lupus enteritis were listed as rare events and were determined from published case reports. Lupus enteritis is described as a vasculitis of the vessels supplying the intestines and is linked to a high acuity SLE score.[22]

Rheumatoid arthritis and gastrointestinal organs
RA is a systemic AD and is one of the most frequently occurring ADs present in 1% of the population of North America and Europe. GI complications directly attributed to RA are found in chronic patients who are undiagnosed or not participating in a suppression medical regimen. RA has generalized inflammation due to self-reactive T and B lymphocytes that release a cascade of activated cytokines.[23] Upper GI involvement is due to temporomandibular joint inflammation and atlantoaxial subluxation. The jaw is swollen making chewing painful and difficult. The cervical one joint has frozen in place making food movement to the esophagus difficult because of the limited of range of motion. This limitation results in dysphagia and dysmotility. Additionally, the pancreas exocrine functions may be impaired because of secondary Sjögren syndrome. Sjögren syndrome is a condition that is often a dual finding with an AD. This syndrome is characterized by a diminished production of all exocrine secretions, such as tears, salivation, and vaginal lubrication. With the decreased digestive enzyme secretion, the breakdown of carbohydrates, fats, and proteins is diminished. RA also promotes an acceleration of atherosclerosis, and cytokine stimulation may lead to the

development of vasculitis.[23] This vasculitis reduces blood flow to the GI tract and leads to abdominal pain and intestinal perforation. RA-associated vasculitis may be a cofactor in gastric and duodenal ulceration as well. Vasculitis of the arteries of the colon from RA may be confused with a presentation of UC. Felty syndrome is a rare RA-associated critical illness that is associated with a state of highly destructive cytokine activation. The clinical findings of Felty syndrome are nodular RA, spleen enlargement, and leukopenia. The liver enzymes are elevated, and esophageal varices may be present as well. Felty syndrome is a severe and lethal AD.[21]

Autoimmune Disease Pharmacology: Iatrogenic Damage to the Gastrointestinal Tract

Glucocorticoids and NSAID

In autoimmune diseases, the pharmacologic interventions are used to reduce symptoms, relieve pain, improve quality of life, and stop progression of tissue destruction in ADs. However, these interventions also have the potential to create an acute episode of GI illness for patients with ADs. The mainstay of acute AD treatment is glucocorticoids. Glucocorticoids have extensive side effects (**Table 5**). In ADs, the desired actions of glucocorticoids are to reduce the circulating levels of prostaglandins and other proinflammatory cytokines.[24] Stomach prostaglandins have a protective role. A loss of these needed prostaglandins impacts the level of mucus present within the stomach. This gastric mucous layer prevents the hydrochloric acid from producing gastritis, peptic ulcer disease, or gastric bleeding.

Nonsteroidal antiinflammatory drugs (NSAIDs) are often concurrently given with glucocorticoids to relieve the pain-associated inflammation with an ADs. The outcome of the mechanism of action of NSAIDs is that prostaglandin production is also reduced. This reduction leads to platelet dysfunction and sets up for gastric complications, especially gastric bleeding. Glucocorticoids and NSAIDs when given concurrently synergistically increase the risk of a GI bleed. Approximately 16,000 to 17,000 GI bleed deaths are associated with NSAID use in the United States annually. The only reversal agent for the undesirable platelet effects of NSAIDs is platelet transfusions and time. Long-term use of NSAIDs is also associated with renal insufficiency.[23] The renal microcirculation needs beneficial prostaglandins for optimization of blood flow.

Disease-modifying drugs: think liver

Disease-modifying drugs (DMDs) are medications that decrease severity and promote remission periods for patients with ADs. DMDs that have significant GI side effects are

Table 5	
Systemic actions of glucocorticoids administration	
Tissues Impacted	**Side Effects**
Central nervous system and eyes	Depression, insomnia, cataracts, restlessness
Cardiovascular	Hypertension, fluid retention
GI	Peptic ulceration, gastritis, and nausea
Dermatologic	Acne, ecchymosis, fragility, moon face appearance, buffalo hump
Musculoskeletal	Muscle wasting, osteoporosis

Data from Visseren T, Darwish Murad S. Recurrence of primary sclerosing cholangitis, primary biliary cholangitis and auto-immune hepatitis after liver transplantation. Best Pract Res Clin Gastroenterol 2017;31(2):187–98; and Alves S, Fasano S, Isenberg DA. Autoimmune gastrointestinal complications in patients with systemic lupus erythematosus: case series and literature review. Lupus 2016;25:1509–19.

methotrexate and leflunomide. Methotrexate has multiple black box warnings because of its mechanism of action that interferes with folic acid.[24] Folic acid is essential to multiple intercellular chemical events. All organs with rapidly dividing cells, such as the GI tract and bone marrow, are set up for adverse events because of the role of folic acid in cell division. However, methotrexate is often prescribed for RA. Another concern for the GI tract is the impact of methotrexate on the hepatic system. Methotrexate when ingested with other hepatotoxic drugs and alcohol has a higher likelihood of leading to DILI. Dosing, duration, and monitoring of methotrexate is critical to maximize the benefit for patients while diminishing the risks. The DMD leflunomide is beneficial for patients with ADs but needs extensive liver screening because it can quickly promote acute liver failure in patients with preexisting impairment. It is primarily used in patients with refractory ADs.

Biological compounds
Biological compounds are medications that have greatly improved the quality of life of patients with rapidly progressive ADs. Categories are antitumor necrosis drugs, non–tumor necrosis factor (TNF) drugs, and Janus kinase inhibitors. All biological medications produce a state of immunosuppression that must be monitored.[25] Bacterial infections and opportunistic infections are the most serious adverse effects. There are also case reports of GI perforation and pancreatitis as adverse side effects of this AD medication classification. Four different biological compounds that are commonly used in ADs are listed in **Table 6**.

Two Case Illustrations

Listed next are 2 case studies that detail the process of care that can be required in critical care for patients with ADs. The cases are a composite of patients cared for in critical care by the author and are deidentified.

Organ-Specific Autoimmune Disease

A 25-year-old female patient was received from the emergency department with obstructive jaundice, a decreased level of consciousness, elevated serum ammonia, elevated respiratory rate, tachycardia, and liver tenderness and enlargement. The drug screen was negative for alcohol or ingestion of illegal substances. The past medical history was significant for asthma flares with 5 hospitalizations during the last 10 years. Home medications were budesonide (inhaled corticosteroid), zafirlukast

Table 6		
New medication classifications for autoimmune diseases		
Medication	**Classification**	**Mechanism of Action**
Etanercept (Enbrel)	Anti-TNF compound	Binds to TNF making the cytokine inactive
Golimumab (Simponi)	Anti-TNF compound	Binds to TNF making the cytokine inactive
Rituximab (Rituxan)	Monoclonal antibody	Binds to the CD20 antigen on the surface of lymphocytes
Tocilizumab (Actemra)	Interleukin receptor inhibitor	Inhibits interleukin 6, a cytokine of inflammation
Tofacitinib (Xeljanz)	Janus kinase inhibitor	Decreases circulating killer cells, increases B-cell count, and decreases serum C-reactive protein

Data from Refs.[23–25]

(leukotriene inhibitor), and norethindrone (birth control pill). The physical examination revealed bilateral wheezing and positional orthopnea. Arterial blood gases revealed metabolic acidosis and hypoxia. The arterial stick site continued to ooze after the sample was obtained in spite of a pressure dressing. Elective intubation was done without difficulty before transport to an MRI. The MRI revealed surface nodularity, heterogeneous hypoattenuation, and hepatic and spleen enlargement. Abdominal girth was enlarged with ascites and was monitored daily. The intensivist consulted pulmonary and hepatic services. Therapy with steroids was not started for 48 hours until all viral hepatitis laboratory tests, liver biopsy, and extensive immunologic tests could be performed. The patient was started on continuous renal replacement therapy because of an increase in creatinine 24 hours after admission. The nurse noted that the dialysis filter needed to be changed every 12 hours to prevent high pressure in the dialysis circuit. High levels of circulating leukotrienes and immunoglobulins were noted in the immunology assay. Oxygenation was improved quickly by intubation; however, metabolic acidosis persisted into day 6. The hepatologist consulted with the Drug-Induced Liver Injury Network to rule out DILI after hepatitis was ruled out. A tentative diagnosis of AIH was given, and steroids were started and were dosed by weight. The patient showed gradual improvement over a 2-week period. She was extubated when the metabolic acidosis was controlled on day 7. Liver enzymes started declining as steroids were started. The liver biopsy revealed autoantibodies throughout the tissue sample, which confirmed the AD. She was discharged under the care of the liver service, pulmonary service, and rheumatology service.

Systemic Autoimmune Disease with Gastrointestinal Manifestations

A 17-year-old African American girl was admitted from an outlying rural hospital via helicopter for sudden onset of abdominal pain, systemic joint swelling, and pleural effusions. She was obtunded on arrival, and arterial blood gases revealed a severe metabolic acidosis and hypoxia. She groaned through every turn or repositioning. Her orbital areas were swollen shut so that pupil examination was not possible. She had no medical history of a concurrent disease or medication use. Drug and alcohol screen came back negative. No history of a viral or bacterial infection was present. The family history revealed a grandmother with RA, a mother with UC, and a father with sickle cell disease. The patient had the sickle cell trait. Pan cultures and immunologic studies were obtained, and oxygen was started at 100% with a nonrebreather mask. An AE-like swelling of the tongue was noted. The patient was intubated via fiber-optic scope by anesthesia because of the upper airway swelling and lack of cervical mobility. Vasopressors were started to maintain blood pressure, as the systolic pressure decreased to less than 80. An echocardiogram was used to evaluate the fluid status and start normal saline boluses. Because of the low systolic pressure, no dialysis or pheresis could be attempted. At hour 8 of hospitalization, the patient experienced a pulseless electrical activity arrest thought to be due to overwhelming metabolic acidosis. Resuscitation was unsuccessful. The autopsy found multiple organ failure due to extensive microthromboses of the lungs, liver, and kidneys. The patient had high circulating titers of autoantibodies associated with SLE and APS. The cause of death was listed as catastrophic APS.

SUMMARY

ADs associated with the GI tract are chronic diseases that may present acutely in critical care or copresent as a confounding variable in other acute illnesses. Understanding the distinctive needs of patients with ADs through the lens of complex cytokine cascades can lead to a more individualized plan of care. Interventions are directed to the reduction of symptoms and cytokine production. The medication classifications used in ADs may lead to GI tissue destruction as well. Each clinical presentation of acute ADs is distinct and requires that an interdisciplinary team work together to promote optimal clinical outcomes.

REFERENCES

1. Sun J, Chang EB. Exploring gut microbes in human health and disease: pushing the envelope. Genes Dis 2014;1(2):132–9.
2. Autoimmune statistics. AARDA Web site. Available at: https://www.aarda.org/about-aarda/mission-statement/. Accessed May 20, 2017.
3. Quintero OL, Rojas-Villarraga A, Mantilla RD, et al. Autoimmune diseases in the intensive care unit. An update. Autoimmun Rev 2013;12(3):380–95.
4. Grant CR, Liberal R. Liver immunology: how to reconcile tolerance with autoimmunity. Clin Res Hepatol Gastroenterol 2017;41(1):6–16.
5. Gonzalez HC, Jafri S, Gordon SC. Management of acute hepatotoxicity including medical agents and liver support systems. Clin Liver Dis 2017;21(1):163–80.
6. European Association for the Study of the Liver. EASL clinical practice guidelines: autoimmune hepatitis. J Hepatol 2015;63(4):971–1004.
7. Dyson JK, Webb G, Hirschfield GM, et al. Unmet clinical need in autoimmune liver diseases. J Hepatol 2015;62(1):208–18.
8. Vallerand AH, Sanoski CA. Davis drug guide. 15th edition. Philadelphia: F.A. Davis; 2017.
9. Visseren T, Darwish Murad S. Recurrence of primary sclerosing cholangitis, primary biliary cholangitis and auto-immune hepatitis after liver transplantation. Best Pract Res Clin Gastroenterol 2017;31(2):187–98.
10. Corrigan M, Hirschfield GM. Primary biliary cirrhosis. Medicine 2015;43(11): 645–7.
11. Rust C, Beuers U. Medical treatment of primary biliary cirrhosis and primary sclerosing cholangitis. Clin Rev Allergy Immunol 2005;28(2):135–45. Available at: http://www.ncbi.nlm.nih.gov/pubmed/15879619.
12. Valero Liñán AS, Rueda Martínez JL, González Masiá JA, et al. Autoimmune pancreatitis or pancreatic cancer? Cir Esp 2016;94(7):415–7.
13. Small AJ, Loftus CG, Smyrk TC, et al. A case of IgG4-associated cholangitis and autoimmune pancreatitis responsive to corticosteroids. Nat Clin Pract Gastroenterol Hepatol 2008;5(12):707–13.
14. Schneider A, Michaely H, Rückert F, et al. Diagnosing autoimmune pancreatitis with the unifying-autoimmune-pancreatitis-criteria. Pancreatology 2017;17(3): 381–94.
15. Malhotra A, Mandip KC, Shaukat A, et al. All-cause hospitalizations for inflammatory bowel diseases: can the reason for admission provide information on inpatient resource use? A study from a large veteran affairs hospital. Mil Med Res 2016;3(1):28. Available at: http://www.ncbi.nlm.nih.gov/pubmed/27602233.
16. Collins-Yoder AS. Angioedema: clinical presentations and pharmacological management. Dimens Crit Care Nurs 2016;35(4):181–9.
17. Bork K. Angioedema. Immunol Allergy Clin North Am 2014;34(1):23–31. Available at: http://www.ncbi.nlm.nih.gov/pubmed/24262687.
18. Mutnuri S, Khan A, Variyam EP. Visceral angioedema: an under-recognized complication of angiotensin-converting enzyme inhibitors. Postgrad Med

2015;127(2):215–7. Available at: http://search.ebscohost.com/login.aspx?direct=true&db=rzh&AN=109703988&site=ehost-live.

19. Giannakopoulos B, Krilis SA. The pathogenesis of the antiphospholipid syndrome. N Engl J Med 2013;368(11):1033–44.

20. Dempsey AC. Autoimmune diseases and their effect on the GI tract...SGNA's 37th annual course, April 30-May 5, 2010, Orlando, Florida. Gastroenterol Nurs 2010;33(2):151.

21. Alves S, Fasano S, Isenberg DA. Autoimmune gastrointestinal complications in patients with systemic lupus erythematosus: case series and literature review. Lupus 2016;25:1509–19.

22. Shizuma T. Clinical characteristics of concomitant systemic lupus erythematosus and primary biliary cirrhosis: a literature review. J Immunol Res 2015;2015:1–9. Available at: http://search.proquest.com/docview/1684439807.

23. Cafardi JM, Rakatansky H, Alarcón GS. Chapter 10 gastrointestinal manifestations of rheumatoid arthritis. In: Handbook of systemic autoimmune diseases, vol. 8. New York: Elsevier Science & Technology; 2017. p. 333–48. Available at: http://www.sciencedirect.com/science/article/pii/S1571507807000104.

24. Alijotas-Reig J, Esteve-Valverde E, Ferrer-Oliveras R. Treatment with immunosuppressive and biologic drugs of pregnant women with systemic rheumatic or autoimmune disease. Med Clin (Barc) 2016;147(8):352–60.

25. Willrich MAV, Murray DL, Snyder MR. Tumor necrosis factor inhibitors: clinical utility in autoimmune diseases. Transl Res 2015;165(2):270–82. Available at: http://www.ncbi.nlm.nih.gov/pubmed/25305470.

Nutrition Options in Critical Care Unit Patients

Teresa D. Welch, EdD, RN, NEA-BC

KEYWORDS

- Nutrition • Critical care • Intensive care • Enteral feeding • Parenteral feeding
- Prepyloric • Postpyloric • Early feeding

KEY POINTS

- The general state of the body depends largely on it nutritional state; feed critical care unit patients as early as clinically possible.
- Enteral feedings provide the best nutritional options and the best patient outcomes.
- Nursing considerations for prepyloric enteral nutrition.
- Nursing considerations for postpyloric enteral nutrition.
- Nursing considerations for parenteral nutrition.

INTRODUCTION

The general state of the body and how well it works depends largely on how well it is fed. Good nutrition and the significant impact that it has on hospitalized patients cannot be overestimated. In the critical care units (CCU) the significance of good nutrition becomes even more urgent and impactful as the body's demand for nutritional support exponentially increases. The body, under stress of critical illness, is working to maintain its basic metabolic functions while also working to build and rebuild tissue in a hypermetabolic state.[1] According to the Society of Critical Care Medicine and the American Society for Parenteral and Enteral Nutrition (ASPEN), "critical illness is typically associated with a catabolic stress state in which patients commonly demonstrate a systemic inflammatory response"[1] often leading to infection, organ dysfunction, and increased morbidity and mortality.[1–4] Research has shown that nutritional support lessens metabolic changes associated with critical illness[3,5,6] and improves the body's ability to respond to medical interventions.[5]

Despite overwhelming evidence to support the significant impact of nutritional therapy in the CCU, "22% to 43% of critically ill patients remain underfed and malnourished."[2,7] In a collaborative effort to address inconsistent feeding practices in

Disclosure Statement: The author reports no real or perceived vested interests that relate to this article that could be construed as a conflict of interest.
Capstone College of Nursing, The University of Alabama, Box 870358, 601 University Boulevard East, Tuscaloosa, AL 35401, USA
E-mail address: tdwelch@ua.edu

Crit Care Nurs Clin N Am 30 (2018) 13–27
https://doi.org/10.1016/j.cnc.2017.10.002

CCUs, Society of Critical Care Medicine and ASPEN have developed evidence-based practice guidelines for timely nutritional assessments and nutritional support that promote optimal patient outcomes.[1] These guidelines recommend (1) early nutritional assessments to identify potential and/or at-risk patients for malnutrition within 12 hours of CCU admission, (2) the initiation of tube feeding access, and (3) enteral nutrition (EN) feeding within the first 24 to 48 hours of admission (**Table 1**).[1,3,8]

NUTRITIONAL OPTIONS

Few critically ill patients are able to tolerate oral intake while in CCU. The delivery of nutritional support should be an interprofessional collaborative effort[2] led by the patient's primary caregiver. Nurses play an integral role in identifying patients at nutritional risk[2] and coordinating the interprofessional team. The interprofessional nutritional support team involves many health care professionals specializing in nutritional therapy, including but not limited to, the critical care nurse, clinical dieticians, and physicians.[2,3] These professionals assess the patient to determine nutritional requirements, prescribe appropriate nutritional therapy, and ensure proper delivery of therapy while mitigating potential complications.[2,3]

Critical care nurses are responsible for the on-going assessment, management, and evaluation of the patient as enteral or parenteral feedings are initiated. Patients must be monitored closely for signs and symptoms of intolerance and/or potential complications.[2,3] As the patient's primary caregiver, the critical care nurse is well positioned to influence and implement evidence-based nutritional practice (**Box 1**).[2]

The ultimate goal for nutritional therapy is to provide the critically ill patient with sufficient nutritional intake to meet the hypermetabolic demands of critical illness. Nutritional therapy in the CCU typically bypasses the oral cavity to deliver feedings directly into the gastrointestinal (GI) tract or vascular system.[1,3,9] Therapeutic decisions related to timing, route, and type of feeding are based on patients underlying nutritional states at the onset of acute illness, the nature of the disease process, severity of the illness, and comorbidities.[1,3,4,8]

EN is the process of providing nutrition directly to the GI tract using an enteral access device (EAD).[9] EN may be delivered prepyloric directly to the stomach or postpyloric directly into the small bowel. Parenteral nutrition (PN) is the process of providing nutritional therapy directly to the circulatory system by way of a peripheral or central venous access device when GI feedings are not feasible.[10]

ENTERAL ROUTE

"If the gut works, use it!"[11] Enteral nutritional therapy is the feeding method of choice in critically ill adult patients when they still maintain a functional GI tract but are unable to swallow or take in sufficient amounts of nutrients by mouth.[1–4,7,9,12–20] Administering EN feedings directly into the GI tract supports normal digestive processes, helps to restore intestinal motility, reduces the stress response, and maintains GI integrity and function while supporting immunity, and minimizing the translocation of bacteria and other organisms. Early EN feedings improve wound healing, decrease the incidence of infection, and decrease hospital length of stay.[1,3,7,9,12]

The nurse is responsible for selecting the appropriate EAD when EN is initiated based on the prescribed formula, anticipated duration of therapy, anatomic considerations presented by the patient, and the current clinical status of the patient.[2,9] Two types of enteral tubes are commonly used in CCU: prepyloric (gastric) tubes and postpyloric (small bowel) feeding tubes. The tip of the prepyloric tube should remain in the stomach above the pyloric sphincter. These

Table 1
Critical care nutrition guidelines

Management of Feeding	
Route	Recommend EN over PN in critically ill patients.
Initiate EN	Recommend early nutritional support therapy within 24–48 h of admission in the patient who cannot maintain adequate intake on their own.
Use of protocols	Recommend development and implementation of EN feeding protocols to increase percentage of nutritional goals met.
Initiate PN	Initiate PN on admission for patients at high nutritional risk or severely malnourished when EN is not feasible. Recommend EN supplementation with PN after 7–10 d if unable to meet >60% of energy and protein needs with EN alone.
Hold PN	In patients presenting low nutritional risk hold PN for 7 d following CCU admission for the patient who cannot maintain adequate intake on their own or receive EN.
Gastric residuals	Recommend patients be monitored for EN intolerance. Inappropriate cessation of EN is avoided. Avoid withholding EN for GRV <500 mL in the absence of other signs of intolerance.
Risk of aspiration	Patients should be assessed for risk of aspiration and proactive measures undertaken to decrease risk. • Recommend postpyloric feeding for those patients who are at high risk for aspiration or not tolerating gastric EN • Elevate head of bed 30°–45°, unless contraindicated. • Recommend continuous feedings rather than bolus feedings • Chlorahexidine mouthwash twice daily. • Recommend prokinnetic agents be initiated in patients at high risk for aspiration.
Placement confirmation	• Gold standard: radiologic confirmation after initial placement and before instillation of medication or feedings. • Capnography • pH <5 indicates gastric content • In adults do not rely on auscultory methods of confirmation • Mark the exit of the tube at the time of placement • DO NOT REPLACE MALPOSITIONED NGT AFTER GASTRECTOMY
Flush and irrigation	• Use distilled or sterile water for flushing and hydration of the immunocompromised patient. • Flush with 30–100 mL of water every 4–6 h during continuous feeding or before and after intermittent feedings. • Flush the tube with 30 mL water after measurement of GRV. • Flush with 30 mL of water before and after medications (follow hospital policy and procedure related to medication administration).

Abbreviations: GRV, gastric residual volume; NGT, nasogastric tube; PN, parenteral nutrition.

Data from Marshall AP, Cahill NE, Gramlich L, et al. Optimizing nutrition in intensive care units: empowering critical care nurses to be effective agents of change. Am J Crit Care 2012;21(3):187–94; and McClave SA, Martindale RG, Vanek VW, et al. Guidelines for the provision and assessment of nutrition support therapy in the adult critically ill patient: Society of Care Medicine (SCCM) and American Society for Parenteral and Enteral Nutrition (A.S.P.E.N.). JPEN J Parenter Enteral Nutr 2009;33(3):277–316.

types of tubes are preferred for intermittent feeding and support gastric absorption. The tip of the postpyloric feeding tube is placed beyond the stomach and pyloric sphincter in the proximal duodenum or jejunum distal to the ligament of Treitz (**Table 2**).[17]

Box 1
The nurse's role in managing EN therapy

- Assess the patient's nutritional status on admission.
- Assess barriers to initiate feeding.
- Collaborate as an active member of an interdisciplinary team focused on meeting the patient's nutritional requirements.
- Assess/minimize barriers to meeting established nutritional therapy goals once feedings have begun.
- Incorporate nutrition as a therapeutic priority of care rather than an adjunctive therapy.
- Minimize interruptions in feedings.
- Assess, and reassess for potential complications associated with nutritional therapy.

Data from Marshall AP, Cahill NE, Gramlich L, et al. Optimizing nutrition in intensive care units: empowering critical care nurses to be effective agents of change. Am J Crit Care 2012;21(3):187–94.

Prepyloric Tubes

Nasogastric and orogastric tubes

Enteral access may be acquired in one of three ways: (1) nasal or oral route (nasogastric tube [NGT], orogastric tube [OGT]), (2) percutaneous endoscopic route (percutaneous endoscopic gastrostomy), and (3) surgical or endoscopic route (gastrostomy or jejunostomy).[4]

When the administration of EN is expected to be less than 30 days, the NGT or small bowel feeding tube is preferred over endoscopic or surgically placed gastrostomy or jejunostomy tubes.[4,12,17] There are significant advantages to placing an NGT/OGT when enteral access is needed:

- Placement is typically uncomplicated requiring little expertise[17,21]
- Generally well tolerated by patients
- Readily accessible and do not require additional support for successful placement[17,21]
- Feedings may be started once appropriate placement of the distal tip is verified[17,21]

An NGT/OGT is made of flexible silicon or a polyvinyl chloride plastic material providing access to the stomach through the nose or mouth. The two most common NGT/OGT chosen in CCU are the Levin and Salem Sump.[22] Levin is a single-lumen tube specifically designed for enteral feedings to the stomach. Salem Sump is a dual-lumen tube designed for safe gastric decompression, continuous suction, or gastric feeding.[22]

The Salem Sump is the preferred tube for gastric decompression and is often placed in emergency departments and operating rooms to evacuate the stomach. It is made of a polyvinyl chloride material and has a radiopaque line that extends the length of the tube. The Salem Sump has graduated markings every 10 cm, with a total length of 120 cm ranges and ranges in size from 14F catheter (smaller) to 18F catheter (larger). The two-lumen design safely allows for continuous or intermittent gastric suction or gastric feedings. When the Salem Sump is used for suction the smaller blue lumen vents the tube to atmospheric pressure reducing the risk of ulceration and trauma to the gastric mucosa because it prevents the development of a vacuum seal between the tip of the tube and the gastric mucosa while under suction.[22]

Table 2
Comparison of enteral feeding tubes

Route	Tube	Benefits	Limitations
Prepyloric (gastric) tubes **Administration of EN is expected to be <30 d**			
Nasal/oral with tip terminating in the stomach	Salem Sump	• Used for gastric decompression, continuous and intermittent suction, or feeding • Dual lumen • Blue side lumen for safety; never kink, tie off, or occlude this port • Radiopaque • Clear polyvinyl chloride, slightly more rigid than comparables • One-way antireflux valve	• Tube is marked to manage depth on insertion; gastric aspirate stains linens; leaks from blue side port
Nasal/oral with tip terminating in the stomach	Levin	• Single lumen • Feeding • No suction	• No radiopaque markings
Nasal/oral with tip terminating in the stomach	Andersen	• Used for gastric decompression, continuous and intermittent suction, or feeding • "If it's bubbling it's working" • Pliable, designed for patient comfort • May come packaged with plastic stylet • Radiopaque • Permanently attached air vent; soft, pliable	• Difficult to insert
Surgical placement with tip terminating in the stomach	Gastrostomy	• Long-term placement >30 d	• Difficult to obtain accurate GRV • Physician to insert • Poses risk of implantation in stomach wall • Poses risk for balloon migration and obstruction of pylorus
Endoscopy placement with tip terminating in stomach	Percutaneous endoscopic gastrostomy tube	• Long-term placement >30 d • Minimally invasive • Allows administration of crushed medications; difficult to obtain accurate GRV • Physician to place	

(continued on next page)

Table 2
(continued)

Route	Tube	Benefits	Limitations
Postpyloric (small bowel) tubes			
Nasal/oral	Dobhoff	• Weighted tip • Small bore; comfortable for patient • Two ports • Comes with wire stylet • Radiopaque • Smaller bore diameter than compared with standard tubes • Tube tends to collapse with suction • Never reinsert the stylet • Must be thoroughly flushed every 4–6 h to prevent clogging • Highly viscous EN formulas clog the tube • Request liquid medications when possible • Time consuming, difficult to insert	• Can be used to provide gastric suction while feeding in the small bowel
Nasal/oral with tip terminating in the proximal duodenum or jejunum	CorPak	• Weighted tip for ease of placement • Ultrasound-guided bedside placement • May be placed by trained registered nurse • Time consuming, difficult to insert, requires skill • Radiopaque	
Nasal/oral	Weighted-magnetized small bowel feeding tubes	• Weighted tip for ease of placement • Magnetized handle • Use magnet and weighted tip to "pull tip forward" • Time consuming, difficult to insert, requires skill • Radiopaque	
Endoscopy or surgery; tip terminates in the small intestine	Jejunal tube	• Terminates in the small intestine • Small bore, single tube • Collapses easily • Clogs easily	

Abbreviation: GRV, gastric residual volume.

The Salem Sump is packaged with a one-way antireflex valve that should be firmly seated in the blue vent lumen (blue tip of the antireflex valve seated into blue lumen). This one-way valve prevents excess gastric fluid from leaking through the blue vent lumen. Do not tie off or otherwise occlude the blue side port lumen for any reason because this disables the safety mechanism of the air vent. If gastric content migrates upward in the blue lumen one may gently clear it by flushing the lumen with air (20 mL) or a small amount (30 mL) of distilled water using a catheter-tipped syringe. Keep the blue lumen well positioned above the level of the patient's waist to minimize gastric content leakage. If the blue antireflex valve becomes wet, the integrity of the valve has been compromised and must be replaced or removed with the lumen left open to air (**Fig. 1**).[7,12,13]

The Levin tube is a single-lumen NGT and depending on the manufacturer may have radiopaque markings to identify the tube on radiographic studies. It has three circular markings strategically located along the length of the tube to help in the process of insertion. The tube is commonly available in sizes 14F catheter (small) to 18F catheter (large) for adults and measures 90 to 110 cm in length. The design of the Levin does not support safe gastric decompression. Caution must be observed if suction is applied using this tube because the negative air pressure can create a vacuum along the stomach wall (if the proximal tip of the tube rests against tissue) and injure the stomach lining through trauma or erosion (**Fig. 2**).[22]

The Anderson tube is a highly flexible medical-grade vinyl tube engineered with the patient's comfort in mind. Because of the pliability of the Andersen tube some models are packaged with a plastic stylet to assist with insertion. It has a radiopaque line that courses the length of the tube. Like the Salem Sump, the Andersen tube has a double-lumen design that prevents vacuum ulceration of gastric mucosa. It is packaged with a permanently attached antireflex valve that eliminates the migration of gastric secretions up the vent lumen. The Andersen tube has a uniquely configured aspiration port designed to reduce tube maintenance and irrigation. Andersen's claim to fame is, "If it's bubbling it's working," providing visible proof of effective suction (**Fig. 3**).[23,24]

Gastrostomy tube and percutaneous esophageal gastrostomy tube

A gastrostomy tube is surgically or endoscopically placed by a physician through the abdominal wall directly into the stomach bypassing the mouth and esophagus. These types of feeding tubes typically have internal and external bolsters, known as "discs" or "bumpers," to prevent inward/outward migration.[9,15,21] These tubes are placed when the patient is expected to require long-term EN feedings, typically greater

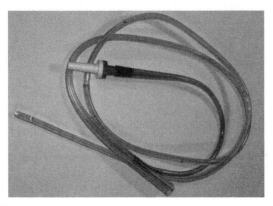

Fig. 1. Salem Sump.

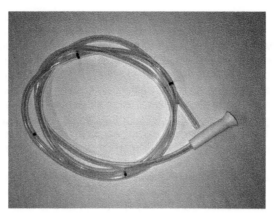

Fig. 2. Levin tube.

than 6 weeks.[12,15] It is important to keep the insertion site clean. The external portion of the G-tube should be secured with tape and covered with gauze to protect the stoma site and prevent displacement of the tube by internal peristaltic migration and possible pyloric obstruction (**Fig. 4**).[12,15]

Postpyloric Feeding Tubes

Duodenal or jejunal small bowel feeding tubes

A postpyloric feeding tube is an enteral feeding device placed surgically/endoscopically by a physician or inserted and advanced nasally by a trained nurse to the small bowel. The distal tip of the tube is placed in the proximal duodenum or jejunum just past the ligament of Treitz. Postpyloric EN is the preferred route of feeding for patients who have shown intolerance to gastric feedings and/or are at risk for gastric reflux and aspiration.[1,12,17–19,21] These tubes are considered for patients who are expected to require EN feedings for more than 30 days.[4] Small bowel feeding tubes are generally smaller in diameter than gastric tubes ranging in size from 8F catheter to 12F catheter, and are 109 cm to 139 cm in length. They are packaged with a wire guidewire to facilitate placement into the stomach and have a weighted tip to promote passive migration through the pyloric sphincter with peristaltic motion.[19] Small bowel feeding tubes are typically made of a radiopaque polyurethane material, and because of their small

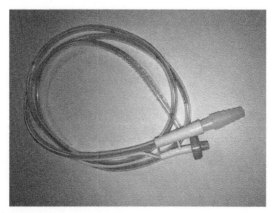

Fig. 3. Andersen tube.

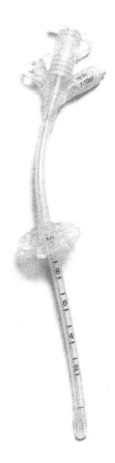

Fig. 4. G- tube.

size and pliability occlude easily and collapse under suction.[19] Placing a nasoenteric, small bowel feeding tube, may be technically challenging at the bedside, and requires specialized training, equipment, and expertise for insertion (**Fig. 5**).[17]

Management of Nasogastric and Orogastric Tubes

Verify placement

After the EAD is placed the gold standard[9,15] for confirming correct tip placement is the interpreted radiograph that visualizes the entire tube.[2,9,12,21] Confirmation of tip placement must be reassessed every 4 hours and before instillation of feedings, hydration, or medications.[9,12,21] Observation for signs and symptoms of respiratory distress during EAD insertion is important, but the lack of signs and symptoms of respiratory distress may not be an indication of appropriate placement of the tube.[1,2,9] The auscultory method of tip placement verification has proven to be an unreliable assessment tool in the determination of tip placement and should not be used.[1,4,9,12,14,21,22,25] Evidence-based recommendations for EAD tip reassessment and placement confirmation are any two of the following measures[25]:

- Mark and document EAD length noted numerically or by marking at the exit site of the tube on insertion and reassessed every 4 hours or before being accessed. If migration is suspected obtain repeat radiograph.[1,2,9,25]

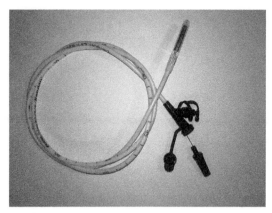

Fig. 5. Small bowel feeding tube.

- Evaluate whether the incremental marking or external tube length changes.[1,2,9,14,15,21,25]
- Capnography (CO_2 sensing).[14,25]
- Obtain a tube aspirate for appearance and pH measurement. Fasting gastric aspirates are typically clear and colorless or green or brown with a pH less than or equal to 5.[9,14,25]

Flush and irrigation

To maintain patency of the EAD it is recommended that the device be flushed every 4 to 6 hours with 30 mL to 100 mL of sterile water. The larger the flush volume, the more effective at maintaining tube patency; however, the amount of water used in a flush must take into account the patient's fluid needs and restrictions.[2,9] Because of the small diameter of postpyloric tubes routine flushing with water is imperative to prevent clogs.[17] Evidence-based recommendations for flushing EADs include the following:

- Sterile water is considered best practice to flush EADs or to hydrate the immunocompromised patient.[2,9]
- Flush the gastric feeding tube with 30 mL distilled water after measurement of gastric residual volume (GRV) in an adult patient.[9]
- Sodium chloride concentrations should never be used to flush EADs, dilute or reconstitute medications or hydrate patients unless specifically prescribed by a licensed independent practitioner to treat underlying metabolic or electrolyte disorder.[2,9]
- Store 60-mL catheter tip syringes in a clean dry fashion as two pieces (piston being removed from the barrel of the syringe before storage).[9]

Gastric residual volume

ASPEN guidelines recommend that GRVs are checked every 4 to 6 hours[9,12,25] and the device should be flushed with a minimum of 30 mL of sterile water afterward.[9] As a single assessment finding, elevated residual volumes have little clinical value. Only when combined with other findings do they become significant[9] because they may indicate other underlying problems manifested through delayed gastric emptying.[1,2,4,9] It is not recommended to withhold EN feedings with GRV 250 mL to 500 mL. Volumes less than 500 mL do not increase the incidence of regurgitation, aspiration, or pneumonia.[1,2,4,9] Avoid holding EN feedings for GRVs less than 500 mL in the absence of other signs of intolerance.[1,2,4,9,12]

Minimize interruptions to enteral nutrition

When managing EN feedings the focus of the critical care nurse is to meet the established nutritional goals of the patient and to assess for and manage potential complications related to EN feedings.[3] It is important to strategically plan nursing care to minimize periods of nothing-by-mouth status before, during, and after diagnostic tests or procedures preventing inadequate delivery of nutrients and possible ileus.[1] So long as the patient remains hemodynamically stable, it is safe and appropriate to feed the patient with mild to moderate ileus. EN promotes gut motility and it is safe to initiate EN feedings before the emergence of overt signs of GI function, such as bowel sounds, the passage of flatus, or stool.[1]

PARENTERAL ROUTE

PN is the process of providing nutritional therapy directly to the circulatory system via peripheral or central venous access device when GI feedings are not feasible.[1,4,10,11,26] According to ASPEN and the European Society for Clinical Nutrition and Metabolism guidelines, when adequate nutritional support cannot be achieved through the GI tract or is not a viable or feasible option for patients, the potential risks and complications of PN therapy no longer outweigh the therapeutic benefits of PN.[1,10,13] PN is an intravenous admixture specifically formulated to meet the specific nutritional needs of the patient. It is given directly into the bloodstream through an intravenous catheter[1,26] The osmolarity, pH, and chemical formulation of the PN admixture determine the intravenous route of administration to a peripheral access (ie, antecubital fossa) or central access (ie, inferior vena cava) catheter.[11] Severity of illness and underlying nutritional status determine the appropriate time to introduce PN support. If there is evidence of malnutrition on admission and EN is not feasible, it is appropriate to initiate PN as soon as possible following admission, resuscitation, and stabilization.[1,26] By contrast, for those individuals who were healthy and well-nourished before the onset of critical illness PN should not be initiated until the seventh day of hospitalization following stabilization of electrolyte imbalances **(Table 3)**.[1,10,11,26]

Peripheral Administration

The role of peripheral PN (PPN) is limited by an increased risk for phlebitis because of the hyperosmolar nature of the formulas.[10,11] Despite having lower concentrations of nutrients when compared with central admixtures of PN, PPN formulas continue to have osmolarity values greater than 600 mOsm/L.[11] PPN admixtures should not be used if the osmolarity exceeds 850 mOsm/L.[20] PPN therapy is indicated for short-term use (<14 day) as a "bridge therapy during transition periods"[11] when oral enteral intake is suboptimal or circumstances exist that do not justify placing a central venous catheter (CVC).[11] The administration of PPN through short cannulas or midline catheters has major limitations in the availability of peripheral veins. They also pose an increased risk of peripheral vein thrombophlebitis requiring careful surveillance for potential signs and symptoms of complications **(Box 2)**.[11,20]

Central Administration

Central admixtures of PN are also known as total PN (TPN)[10] and have the capacity to provide complete nutrition.[10,11] The administration of TPN should only be considered

Table 3
Comparison of peripheral and central total parenteral nutrition

Advantages	Disadvantages
Enteral	
• Physiologic • Simpler • Less expensive • No central venous catheter required for administration • Less invasive • Less monitoring • Less complications	• Requires functional GI tract • Diarrhea • Aspiration • Intolerance formula • Malposition of tubes • Sinusitis
Parenteral	
• Does not require functional GI tract • Provides total parenteral nutrition (central formula)	• Nonphysiologic: GI tract atrophies with prolonged use • Requires venous access • Increased risk of systemic infection • Increased risk of pneumothorax • Routine (daily) monitoring of laboratory studies • Expensive • Potential for more complications

for patients who meet specific medical conditions[13,20] when EN is not a feasible option and therapy is expected to last more than 7 days.[1] TPN formulas are hyperosmolar concentrations that because of their high osmolarity require central venous access for rapid dilution within the high blood flow rates of central circulation.[10,20] The tip of the CVC should optimally be located in the lower third of the superior vena cava, or the upper portion of the right atrium where blood flow rates are sufficient to rapidly dilute the hypertonic feeding formulation.[10,20]

Complications caused by TPN are typically associated with either the catheter access device or the pharmaceutical admixture.[10] Central venous access is critical to the delivery of TPN, yet access devices are a leading source of complications associated with TPN therapy, most notably central line–associated bloodstream

Box 2
Evidence-based interventions for the prevention of peripheral vein thrombophlebitis

- Aseptic technique for catheter placement and catheter care.[20,27]
- Choice of smallest gauge possible (ideally the diameter of the catheter should be one-third or less of the diameter of the vein, as checked by ultrasound).[20]
- Short-term use.
- Use of polyurethane or silicone catheters.[20]
- Osmolarity of solution <850 mOsm/L.[20]
- Use of lipid-based solutions.[20]
- pH of solution >5 or <9.[20]
- Develop standardized insertion and management protocols for intravenous therapy.

Data from Pittiruti M, Hamilton H, Biffi R, et al. ESPEN guidelines on parenteral nutrition: central venous catheters (access, care, diagnosis and therapy of complications). Clin Nutr 2009;28:365–77; and U.S. Department of Health and Human Services. Agency for Healthcare Research and Quality (AHRQ). CLABSI Tools. 2014. Available at: https://www.ahrq.gov/professionals/education/curriculum-tools/clabsitools/index.html. Accessed June 12, 2017.

infections. Because TPN recipients are often malnourished, immunocompromised, and require intravenous therapy for extended periods of time, they are particularly high risk for central line–associated bloodstream infections.[11]

CVC access devices are classified based on anticipated duration of use (short term, midterm, and long term). Most hospitalized patients have a short-term CVC access device placed if central access is warranted and the anticipated need is less than 30 days. These devices may be single-lumen or multilumen nontunneled catheters measuring 20 cm to 30 cm in length. They are placed in the subclavian, internal jugular, innominate, or axillary vein with the tip advanced to the superior vena cava, or upper portion of the right atrium for central access.[20] Midterm central catheters are usually nontunneled CVC access devices intended for intermittent use up to 3 months.[20] These types of catheters are typically single- or dual-lumen devices 50 cm to 60 cm long. They are peripherally inserted into the basilic, brachial, or cephalic vein with the tip advanced to the superior vena cava, or upper portion of the right atrium for central access.[20] Peripherally inserted central catheters are an example of midterm catheters used in acute care. Long-term access devices are typically cuffed tunneled (implantable) Hickman, Groshong, or Broviac catheters surgically placed for patients requiring CVC access greater than 3 months (**Box 3**).[20]

Box 3
Evidence-based recommendations for management of TPN

Catheter

- Adequate hand washing policy.
- CVC access.
- Less than 30 days.
- Prevention of catheter-associated complications.
  - Follow evidence-based central line–associated bloodstream infection guidelines or bundles promoted by the Institute of Healthcare Improvement
  - Postprocedural radiologic confirmation of CVC tip placement is required for all CVC insertions where the position of the tip was not verified during the procedure
  - Avoid femoral, neck, antecubital fossa sites for insertion because they have higher risk of contamination

Admixture

- Aseptic technique.
- Verify TPN order and inspect admixture for particulate matter before administration.
- Change IV tubing every 24 hours when using TPN or every 72 hours if lipids are not used.
- Administer via IV pump through a dedicated, labeled IV line.
- In-line filters do not prevent catheter-related bloodstream infection. Follow pharmacist's recommendations for in-line filter use related to filtering miroaggregates possibly occurring in lipid-based TPN solutions.
- Obtain baseline laboratory work; serum glucose, complete metabolic profile, CBC, and liver profile
  - Monitor serial blood glucose every 6 hours
  - Monitor weekly complete metabolic profile, CBC
  - Monitor daily weights
  - Liver function test biweekly

Abbreviations: CBC, complete blood count; IV, intravenous.
  Data from Refs.[11,13,20]

SUMMARY

Critically ill patients have increased metabolic requirements and must rely on the administration of nutritional feedings to meet increased demands.[1–4] Yet, according to research almost half of all hospitalized patients are not fed, are underfed, or are malnourished while in the hospital.[7] This article demonstrates available resources open to nurses enabling them to initiate and manage early feedings to meet the nutritional needs of the patient. EN has proven to be an important therapeutic strategy for improving the outcomes of critically ill patients, and the critical care nurse plays an integral role in their success.[2]

REFERENCES

1. McClave SA, Martindale RG, Vanek VW, et al. Guidelines for the provision and assessment of nutrition support therapy in the adult critically ill patient: Society of Care Medicine (SCCM) and American Society for Parenteral and Enteral Nutrition (A.S.P.E.N.). JPEN J Parenter Enteral Nutr 2009;33(3): 277–316.
2. Marshall AP, Cahill NE, Gramlich L, et al. Optimizing nutrition in intensive care units: empowering critical care nurses to be effective agents of change. Am J Crit Care 2012;21(3):187–94.
3. O'Leary C, Bawel-Brinkley K. Nutrition support protocols: enhancing delivery of enteral nutrition. Crit Care Nurse 2017;37(2):15–23.
4. Miller KR, Kiraly LN, Lowen CC, et al. "CAN WE FEED": a mnemonic to merge nutrition and intensive care assessment of the critically ill patient. JPEN J Parenter Enteral Nutr 2011;35(5):643–59.
5. Cherry-Bukowiec JR. Optimizing nutrition therapy to enhance mobility in critically ill patients. Crit Care Nurs Q 2013;36(1):28–36.
6. Alberda C, Gramlich L, Jones N, et al. The relationship between nutritional intake and clinical outcomes in critically ill patients: results of an international multicenter observational study. Intensive Care Med 2009;35(10):1728–37.
7. Stewart ML. Nutrition support protocols and their influence on the delivery of enteral nutrition: a systematic review. Worldviews Evid Based Nurs 2014;11(3): 194–9.
8. DeLegge MH. Nutrition support in the intensive care patient. J Infus Nurs 2013; 36(4):262–8.
9. Boullata JI, Carrera AL, Harvey L, et al. ASPEN Safe practices for enteral nutrition therapy. JPEN J Parenter Enteral Nutr 2017;41(1):15–103.
10. Tilton J. Benefits and risks of parenteral nutrition in patients with cancer. Onc Nur Adv 2011;28–34.
11. Worthington PH, Gilbert KA. Parenteral nutrition: risks, complications, and management. J Infus Nurs 2012;35(1):52–64.
12. Rose K. Nutrition. In: Potter AG, Perry PA, Stockert PA, et al, editors. Fundamentals of nursing. 9th edition. St Louis (France): Elsevier Inc;; 2017. p. 1053–100.
13. Pierre S, Berger MM, Van den Berghe G, et al. ESPEN guidelines on parenteral nutrition: intensive care. Clin Nutr 2009;28:387–400.
14. Flynn-Makic MB, Rauen C, Watson R, et al. Examining the evidence to guide practice: challenging practice habits. Crit Care Nurse 2014;34(2):28–45.
15. Fletcher J. Nutrition: safe practice in adult enteral tube feeding. Br J Nurs 2011; 20(19):1234–9.
16. Elke G, van Zanten ARH, Lemieux M, et al. Enteral versus parenteral nutrition in critically ill patients: an updated systematic review and meta-analysis of

randomized controlled trials. Crit Care 2016;117. https://doi.org/10.1186/s13054-016-1298-1.

17. Jabbar A, McClave SA. Pre-pyloric versus post-pyloric feeding. Clin Nutr 2005; 24:719–26.

18. Jiyong J, Tiancha H, Huiqin W, et al. Effect of gastric versus post-pyloric feeding on the incidence of pneumonia in critically ill patients: observations from traditional and Bayesian random-effects meta-analysis. Clin Nutr 2013;32:8–15.

19. Gokhale A, Kantoor S, Prakash S, et al. Bedside placement of small-bowel feeding tube in intensive care unit for enteral nutrition. Indian J Crit Care Med 2016;26(6):357–60.

20. Pittiruti M, Hamilton H, Biffi R, et al. ESPEN guidelines on parenteral nutrition: central venous catheters (access, care, diagnosis and therapy of complications). Clin Nutr 2009;28:365–77.

21. Hoiston A, Fuldaur P. Enteral feeding: indications, complications, and nursing care. Am Nurse Today 2017;12(1):20–5.

22. Walsh K, Schub E. Nasogastric tube: insertion and verifying placement in adult patient. Glendale (CA): CINAH Information Systems; 2016.

23. Andersen NasogastricTubes. Available at: http://nasogastrictubes.anpro.com/nasogastric_tubes/index.htm. Accessed June 10, 2017.

24. Dobhoff feeding tube. Available at: http://www.medline.com/product/Dobbhoff-Nasogastric-Feeding-Tubes-by-Covidien/Z05-PF10706. Accessed June 10, 2017.

25. Methany N. Practice alert: initial and ongoing verification of feeding tube placement in adults. Crit Care Nurse 2016;36(2):e8–13.

26. Ramakrishnan N, Shankar B, Ranganathan L, et al. Parenteral nutrition support: beyond gut feeling? Quality control study of parenteral nutrition practices in a tertiary care hospital. Indian J Crit Care Med 2016;20(1):36–9.

27. U.S. Department of Health and Human Services. Agency for Healthcare Research and Quality (AHRQ). CLABSI Tools. 2014. Available at: https://www.ahrq.gov/professionals/education/curriculum-tools/clabsitools/index.html. Accessed June 12, 2017.

Mesenteric Ischemia

Robin M. Lawson, DNP

KEYWORDS

- Acute mesenteric ischemia • Chronic mesenteric ischemia • Arterial embolism
- Arterial thrombosis • Mesenteric venous thrombosis
- Nonocclusive mesenteric ischemia

KEY POINTS

- Mesenteric ischemia is an uncommon disease most often seen in the elderly and is classified as either acute or chronic.
- Mesenteric ischemia results from blood flow in the mesenteric circulation that inadequately meets metabolic demands of visceral organs and can lead to bowel wall necrosis.
- Vague symptoms, comorbid conditions, and diagnostic or management delays contribute to extremely high mortalities associated with mesenteric ischemia.
- Computed tomography angiography is the most accurate diagnostic tool for both types of mesenteric ischemia.
- Revascularization via endovascular therapy is the recommended treatment of symptomatic patients who have not yet developed bowel ischemia or necrosis.

INTRODUCTION

Mesenteric ischemia is an uncommon disease most often seen in the elderly.[1] This disease results from blood flow in the mesenteric circulation that inadequately meets metabolic demands of the visceral organs[2] and, if untreated, eventually leads to necrosis of the bowel wall.[3] Mesenteric ischemia is divided into 2 types: acute mesenteric ischemia (AMI) and chronic mesenteric ischemia (CMI).[3] AMI can be further subdivided into 4 different types: nonocclusive mesenteric ischemia, mesenteric venous thrombosis, arterial thrombosis, and arterial embolism,[1,4] depending on the mechanism of insufficient blood flow (**Fig. 1**).[5] When there is a delay in diagnosing CMI, acute-on-chronic mesenteric ischemia may ensue.[6] Regardless of the cause, early diagnosis of mesenteric ischemia is crucial to avert intestinal necrosis and death.

According to the literature, the mortality for AMI is extremely high,[5] ranging from 60% to 80%.[7] Vague symptoms associated with AMI can lead to delayed diagnosis

Disclosure: The author has no financial interests, affiliations, or conflicts of interest that relate to the publication of this material.
Academic Programs, The University of Alabama, Capstone College of Nursing, 650 University Boulevard, East, Tuscaloosa, AL 35401, USA
E-mail address: rmlawson@ua.edu

Crit Care Nurs Clin N Am 30 (2018) 29–39
https://doi.org/10.1016/j.cnc.2017.10.003
0899-5885/18/© 2017 Elsevier Inc. All rights reserved.

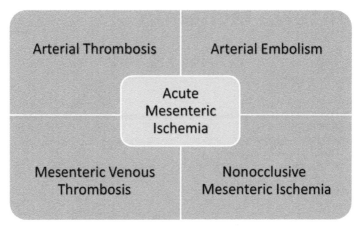

Fig. 1. Types of acute mesenteric ischemia.

and increased mortality.[4,8,9] Diagnostic and management challenges combined with patient comorbidities further contribute to the high mortality.[10] This article highlights recent advances in the early diagnosis and management of mesenteric ischemia that have been shown to be effective in decreasing morbidity and mortality.

PATHOPHYSIOLOGY

Three main arteries comprise the mesenteric circulation: the inferior mesenteric artery (IMA), the celiac trunk, and the superior mesenteric artery (SMA).[11] The celiac trunk predominantly delivers blood to the foregut (stomach and proximal duodenum).[11] The IMA delivers blood to the proximal anal canal, the rectum, the sigmoid and descending colon, and the hindgut (includes distal third of the transverse colon).[11] The SMA delivers blood to the transverse colon (proximal), the ascending colon, the cecum, the small intestine, and the midgut (includes distal duodenum).[11]

The mesenteric vessels are interconnected to adjacent areas by means of collateral vessels.[12] Typically, these vessels accommodate increased perfusion during the postprandial period in order to meet increased physiologic demand during digestion.[11] The ability of the collateral vessels to deliver sufficient blood flow to adjacent areas in times of acute occlusion varies and can be affected by the pattern of occlusion.[12] In acute total occlusion, the collaterals are usually not able to meet the physiologic demands of the gastrointestinal tract.[12,13] An acute single-vessel occlusion, which is usually of the SMA, can lead to profound ischemia very quickly as a result of decreased blood flow through this essential vessel and its collaterals. Because additional collaterals develop over time in CMI, symptoms usually do not develop until 2 or more primary vessels are totally occluded.[2]

ACUTE MESENTERIC ISCHEMIA
Causes

Mesenteric ischemia always occurs secondary to some other type of preexisting disease process.[12] AMI most frequently affects elderly individuals[4,14,15] with numerous atherosclerotic risk factors.[15] The most common causes of AMI are arterial thrombosis and embolism[4,9,16] within the SMA.[9] Nonocclusive mesenteric ischemia is not as common.[1,9] Venous thrombosis represents even fewer cases.[1] Each type of mesenteric ischemia can create a high-risk situation for development of mesenteric infarction and death.[12] Knowledge of identified risk factors and comorbid conditions associated with the different types of AMI can aid in the diagnosis (**Table 1**).

Arterial embolism
Arterial embolism of the SMA is associated with a variety of comorbid conditions. Such conditions include advanced age, smoking, hypertension, cardiac disease,[16,17] hyperlipidemia, diabetes mellitus, and chronic renal insufficiency.[17] Other conditions associated with arterial embolism include ventricular aneurysm, prostatic valve, rheumatic heart disease,[1] atrial fibrillation, and myocardial infarction.[1,12]

Arterial thrombosis
Arterial thrombosis is linked to various identifiable risk factors. These risk factors include hypertension, hyperlipidemia, diabetes, estrogens, arteriosclerosis, and antiphospholipid syndrome.[1] Dehydration,[1,18] hypercoagulable state, and low cardiac output[18] have also been identified as major contributing factors.

Mesenteric venous thrombosis
Mesenteric venous thrombosis is associated with predisposing conditions, such as right-sided heart failure, deep vein thrombosis, cirrhosis, hepatic splenomegaly, sepsis, sickle cell disease,[1] and malignancies.[1,6] Additional conditions associated with mesenteric venous thrombosis are pancreatitis, hepatitis, hypercoagulable disorders,[1,12] portal hypertension,[12] direct abdominal trauma, postoperative state, obesity, and pregnancy.[18]

Nonocclusive mesenteric ischemia
Nonocclusive mesenteric ischemia typically occurs in critically ill patients[1] with low cardiac output[18] brought on by a variety of causes. The final pathway for all causes of this type of mesenteric ischemia is extended intestinal vasoconstriction and decreased intestinal blood flow. Patients with nonocclusive mesenteric ischemia commonly present in a multisystem organ failure/shock state and have historically shown the worst in-hospital mortalities compared with presentations of other types of mesenteric ischemia.[6] Nonocclusive mesenteric ischemia has been shown to occur after cardiopulmonary bypass and is associated with risk factors such as peripheral vascular disease, poor preoperative cardiac state, urgent cardiopulmonary bypass,[14] renal insufficiency,[14,19] diuretic therapy, and age more than 70 years.[19] Longer cardiopulmonary bypass and ventilator times have been shown to be contributing causes.[14] In addition, the need for intra-aortic balloon pump support and inotropic therapy[14] have been identified as serious risk factors.

Independent Risk Factors for Mortality

Additional studies have identified specific independent risk factors for mortality in AMI. Leone and colleagues[5] conducted a multicenter study of 780 cases of AMI to identify independent risk factors for mortality in patients who were admitted to the intensive care unit (ICU). Results showed that advanced age and a sequential organ failure assessment severity score at diagnosis were associated with increased ICU mortality. A plasma lactate level more than 2.7 mmol/L at the time of diagnosis was also an independent risk factor, but a level within the normal range did not eliminate a diagnosis of AMI. The ICU mortality of patients included in this study was 58%, and the in-hospital mortality was 63%.[5]

Akyildiz and colleagues[10] conducted a study to identify factors associated with adverse outcomes in patients diagnosed with AMI. A total of 104 patients were

Table 1
Risk factors for different types of acute mesenteric ischemia

Arterial Embolism	Arterial Thrombosis	Mesenteric Venous Thrombosis	Nonocclusive Mesenteric Ischemia
Advanced age	Hypertension	Right-sided heart failure	Age >70 y
Smoking	Hyperlipidemia	Deep vein thrombosis	Critically ill
Hypertension	Diabetes	Cirrhosis	Low cardiac output
Cardiac disease	Estrogens	Hepatic splenomegaly	Peripheral vascular disease
Hyperlipidemia	Arteriosclerosis	Sepsis	Renal insufficiency
Diabetes mellitus	Antiphospholipid syndrome	Sickle cell disease	Diuretic therapy
Chronic renal insufficiency	Dehydration	Malignancies	Cardiac surgery
Ventricular aneurysm	Hypercoagulable state	Pancreatitis	Poor preoperative cardiac state
Prostatic valve	Low cardiac output	Hepatitis	Urgent and/or extended cardiopulmonary bypass
Rheumatic heart disease		Hypercoagulable disorders	Extended ventilator time
Atrial fibrillation		Portal hypertension	Intra-aortic balloon pump
Myocardial infarction		Direct abdominal trauma	Inotropic therapy
		Postoperative state	
		Obesity	
		Pregnancy	

included. The primary independent factors resulting in poor outcomes were renal insufficiency and the length of necrosis. The 30-day postsurgical mortality was 66.3%. It is possible that these fatal predictors may be prevented with early diagnosis and prompt therapeutic intervention.

Clinical Manifestations

The usual presentation for AMI is an elderly patient with various comorbidities who complains of severe abdominal pain (abdominal angina) out of proportion with that discovered on physical examination.[4] Although pain is the most constant symptom for patients with AMI,[4,16] it is important for health care providers to recognize that the presentation may vary considerably depending on the exact cause.[4] Physical findings that give rise to suspicion of mesenteric ischemia include abdominal distention, abdominal pain, and the presence of peritoneal signs[20] (eg, abdominal guarding, rebound tenderness, and severe abdominal pain worsened by movement). Symptoms may also include vomiting, diarrhea, and hematochezia.[16] Mesenteric venous thrombosis is associated with more insidious symptoms and less extensive disease progression at the time of diagnosis compared with arterial mesenteric ischemia.[18]

Acute abdomen can present diagnostic difficulties for patients with chronic obstruction of the SMA.[15] The chronic obstruction is associated with insidious, rather than acute, onset of symptoms for some patients with AMI. The condition of patients presenting in this manner may deteriorate over several days before the diagnosis is obvious.[15] Premonitory symptoms coupled with a prolonged episode of AMI seems to favor survival.[15]

Diagnosis

An evolution of diagnostic modalities has occurred over the past 20 years.[21] However, early recognition of AMI is still challenging.[22] A high level of suspicion based on the patient's history and the provider's physical examination findings is critical for the accurate diagnosis of AMI.[6] However, this disease cannot be diagnosed based solely on signs and symptoms. Serum laboratory tests are not helpful in establishing a diagnosis either. Therefore, radiologic testing must be performed.[20]

Laboratory tests

Some studies have focused on evaluating the diagnostic accuracy of a variety of serum tests for mesenteric ischemia. Such tests have included D-dimer levels, lactate levels, base excess, leukocyte count, and biomarkers such as alpha-glutathione S-transferase and intestinal fatty acid binding protein (I-FABP).[9] However, there are no serum tests that can be used routinely to accurately diagnose AMI in the early stages.[1,20] Alpha-glutathione S-transferase and I-FABP have been identified as the most promising, but additional research is needed.[1]

Radiologic tests

Because laboratory tests cannot exclude the diagnosis for AMI, clinical suspicion requires evaluation through radiologic tests. Duplex ultrasonography, magnetic resonance angiography, and computed tomography (CT) angiography are radiologic tests that have been used over the years to assess mesenteric vessels.[4,11] A systematic review and meta-analysis conducted by Cudnik and colleagues[20] revealed that the most commonly used and most accurate radiologic test for diagnosing AMI is CT angiography. Other recent studies report that multidetector CT angiography is now the gold standard for diagnosing suspected AMI.[1,9] CT angiography has been shown to be highly sensitive (94%) and specific (95%).[20] Extensive use of this most important and accurate diagnostic tool[1] has been associated with earlier diagnosis and better outcomes for AMI.[12] Not only is CT angiography useful in accurately and rapidly confirming the diagnosis of AMI but it can also identify other conditions, such as the presence of free air, air in the mesenteric vein, peritoneal fluid collection, bowel wall enhancement, and bowel wall thickening.[16] In any situation in which AMI is suspected, especially in elderly patients with a history of cardiovascular disease who report pain that does not match with the physical examination findings, multidetector CT with intravenous contrast should be performed without delay.[1]

Initial Management

As soon as an AMI diagnosis is made, treatment should be instituted immediately[14] to prevent mesenteric infarction, progression of intestinal necrosis, and subsequent death. The European Society for Trauma and Emergency Surgery (ESTES) study group recently published guidelines for the management of AMI based on a systematic review of literature.[1] Initial evidence-based recommendations designed to improve outcomes for the different types of AMI include:

- Arterial embolism and arterial thrombosis: perform endovascular therapy (EVT) whenever possible if bowel necrosis is not evident.[1]
- Venous thrombosis: initiate systemic anticoagulation with low-molecular-weight or unfractionated heparin.[1,2,18] Consider EVT for deteriorating patients.[1]
- Nonocclusive mesenteric ischemia: correct the cause and improve perfusion of the mesentery vasculature via direct vasodilator infusion into the SMA.[1]
- Consider immediate surgery if there is a chance that surgical intervention may be curative for AMI when there is a deterioration in the patient's condition or if signs of peritonitis develop because of bowel necrosis.[1]

Additional key recommendations for managing the severe effects of AMI focus on resuscitation and stabilization of the patient and include the following measures:

- Replenish tissue/organ perfusion with prompt infusion of crystalloids[1,2] and institute immediate supplementary oxygen.[1]
- Avoid vasopressors when possible because the vasoconstrictive effects can further reduce splanchnic perfusion. If a vasopressor is required because of hypovolemia, select one that has little effect on mesenteric blood flow.[1,2]
- Administer broad-spectrum antibiotics during the early stages of AMI to decrease the bacterial translocation that results from reduced integrity of the mucosal barrier.[1,2]
- Consider palliative care only for elderly patients with late presentation and signs of peritonitis or organ failure because of the decreased likelihood of any benefit from invasive procedures.[1]

Revascularization

Both open vascular surgery and EVT approaches to revascularization for the management of AMI have been shown to be effective by observation studies.[18] However, there has been an increase in the use of EVT, which is a minimally invasive procedure.[23] Literature reports that EVT is the best treatment option, especially for patients who are fragile and elderly,[18] those with a poor preoperative condition, and those who have not yet developed bowel ischemia and necrosis.[24] Endovascular techniques used to replenish luminal visceral blood flow include balloon angioplasty, thrombolysis, percutaneous thrombus extraction, and antegrade percutaneous stenting.[14] Such endovascular therapy, including visceral vessel stenting and catheter-directed thrombolysis for AMI, is best performed following early diagnosis before bowel integrity is compromised.[6] Open surgery continues to be the treatment of choice for emergency conditions when bowel ischemia or necrosis is suspected.[24] The following studies highlight recent outcomes in support of EVT for AMI:

- Kärkkäinen and colleagues[15] conducted a study on EVT as a primary revascularization modality in AMI. A total of 58 elderly patients with AMI secondary to thrombotic (32 [64%]) or embolic (18 [36%]) obstruction of the SMA who were referred for revascularization were included. Results showed that EVT was technically successful in 44 (88%) with acceptable EVT-related problems (10%) and complication rates (eg, emergency laparotomy 40%, bowel resection 34%).
- Beaulieu and colleagues[7] compared outcomes of open surgery (OS) and EVT for AMI. The study included a total of 679 patients, whereby 165 (24.3%) had EVT and 514 (75.7%) had OS. Results revealed that revascularization for AMI via EVT, compared with the open approach, was associated with shorter length of stay (12.9 vs 17.1 days), decreased in-hospital mortality (24.9% vs 39.3%), decreased need for bowel resection (14.4% vs 33.4%), and decreased requirement for total parenteral nutrition (13.7% vs 24.4%).
- Zhao and colleagues[24] conducted a systematic review on the management of AMI. A total of 28 articles consisting of 1110 patients undergoing EVT or OS were included in the review. Results indicated that the overall complication rate was significantly lower for the EVT group compared with the OS group. Specifically, the EVT group had decreased rates of myocardial infarction, wound infection, pulmonary infection/failure, and multiple organ dysfunction. In addition, the EVT-specific complication rates (eg, access site bleeding, SMA dissection, and perforation or bleeding) were fairly low.[24]
- Branco and colleagues[23] evaluated the impact of EVT on outcomes for patients with AMI requiring emergency surgical intervention. The EVT-first approach showed decreased risk of death by 2.5-fold, reduced need for laparotomy, decreased transfusion requirements, and diminished complications such as pneumonia and sepsis.

CHRONIC MESENTERIC ISCHEMIA
Causes

CMI is typically caused by occlusion or stenosis of at least 1 of the visceral arteries[25] and occurs most frequently in elderly women[2,26,27] with atherosclerosis[2,26] and a history of smoking.[26] CMI has been linked to cardiovascular risk factors (eg, hypertension, dyslipidemia, and diabetes)[27,28] and comorbidities (eg, history of myocardial infarction, stenting, or coronary bypass), cerebral comorbidities (eg, history of stroke or carotid endarterectomy),[26,28] and renal comorbidity (eg, creatinine clearance lower than 30 mL/min).[28]

Several conditions place hospitalized patients at risk for developing and even dying from CMI. Patients with CMI identified as needing OS and those 70 years of age or older have been shown to be at considerably higher risk for mortality.[29] Li and colleagues[30] found end-stage renal disease (ESRD) to be associated with development of mesenteric ischemia in hospitalized patients. Of the patients included in this study, those undergoing peritoneal dialysis were shown to be at greater risk than those undergoing hemodialysis.[30] Independent risk factors for developing mesenteric ischemia were identified as advanced age, peripheral vascular disease, diabetes, heart failure, atrial fibrillation, neoplasm, pulmonary disease, and peritoneal dialysis[30] (**Table 2**).

Table 2
Conditions associated with chronic mesenteric ischemia

General	Cardiovascular	Cerebral	Renal	Other
Elderly	Hypertension	Stroke	Reduced creatinine	Neoplasm
Female	Dyslipidemia	Carotid	clearance	Pulmonary
Smoking	Diabetes	endarterectomy	ESRD	disease
Atherosclerosis	Myocardial infarction		Hemodialysis	
	Stent placement		Peritoneal dialysis	
	Coronary bypass			
	Atrial fibrillation			

Clinical Manifestations

CMI often includes nonspecific symptoms such as weight loss, postprandial abdominal pain, and food fear.[6,17,21,28] Symptoms may also include early satiety,[17] nausea, vomiting,[6,12,17] diarrhea, and/or bloating after eating.[6] An abdominal bruit may also be present.[12] Because advanced age and a history of smoking are common in patients with CMI, cancer is frequently considered and may lead to a delayed diagnosis.[2] If there is a delay in diagnosis, acute-on-chronic mesenteric ischemia may occur and lead to the development of abdominal guarding, rebound tenderness, and other peritoneal signs as the bowel becomes necrotic with perforation.[6]

Diagnosis

CMI is ultimately a clinical diagnosis made in the context of patient symptoms and anatomic findings.[11] Patients may have mild, transient symptoms of mesenteric atherosclerotic disease and go years without it being recognized before an acute episode of mesenteric ischemia occurs.[26] Conventional angiography and Doppler ultrasonography, both radiologic tests previously used to aid in the diagnosis CMI, have been replaced by CT angiography.[21] Patients with clinical symptoms of splanchnic syndrome (eg, postprandial abdominal pain, weight loss, or food fear) should be highly suspect of CMI and have CT angiography.[21] Mesenteric atherosclerotic disease should be highly suspected in older patients with a history of vascular disease presenting with right-sided colitis that is unexplained.[26] Immediate CT angiography is recommended for patients with known atherosclerotic disease, abdominal pain, *Helicobacter pylori*–negative duodenitis, or right-sided colitis to confirm suspected symptomatic mesenteric atherosclerotic disease.[26]

Revascularization

Treatment of symptomatic CMI is essential to prevent development of AMI, which could lead to mesenteric infarction and death.[13] All patients with CMI who are showing symptoms should undergo revascularization.[2] Endovascular therapy has been performed increasingly for revascularization of CMI over the years with good short-term results.[31] EVT has replaced open revascularization as the preferred treatment of CMI in most centers across the country.[13,29] Recent studies show morbidity rates[21,29] and mortalities[29] to be lower in patients with CMI undergoing EVT compared with those undergoing open revascularization. Stenting is most often used during EVT because angioplasty alone has been shown to be associated with poor patency and unacceptable long-term symptom relief.[2] Covered stents have been used more frequently than bare metal stents in recent years and are associated with less restenosis.[27] The following studies highlight some of the pertinent outcomes related to EVT and effective methods for decreasing the risk of restenosis:

- Cai and colleagues[25] recently conducted a meta-analysis to compare clinical outcomes of open versus endovascular revascularization for CMI. A total of 8 studies with 569 cases (209 EVT cases; 360 OS cases) were included. Results showed a significantly lower in-hospital complication rate and higher recurrence rate within 3 years for endovascular revascularization compared with open revascularization. There was no difference in the 30-day mortality and 3-year cumulative survival rate.
- Grilli and colleagues[17] conducted a study to evaluate the safety and outcomes of EVT for chronic total occlusions of the SMA in patients with CMI. A total of 47 patients who received stents for the occlusions via EVT were included. Results showed excellent clinical outcomes with 95% of the patients free from symptomatic recurrence at 1 year and 78% at 2 years. No major complications were associated with this type of revascularization, and only 3 minor access-related complications occurred.
- AbuRahma and colleagues[13] conducted a long-term study to investigate perioperative and late clinical outcomes of percutaneous transluminal stentings of the superior and celiac mesenteric arteries. A total of 83 patients with CMI who underwent EVT over a 10-year period were included. Of the 83 patients, 54 had SMA stents and 51 had celiac artery stents. Results showed high rates of technical/early clinical success and sufficient long-term clinical outcomes (symptom relief). However, results also showed high rates of late in-stent stenosis, thereby indicating the need for imaging surveillance and reintervention.
- Oderich and colleagues[27] recently compared bare metal stents with covered stents for treatment of chronic atherosclerotic mesenteric arterial disease.[27] A total of 225 patients from one of 2 participating academic centers who received treatment (eg, 164 patients/197 vessels with bare metal stent placement and 61 patients/67 vessels with covered stent placement) were included. Coated stents were associated with lower rates of restenosis, symptom recurrence, and reinterventions compared with bare metal stents.
- Hogendoorn and colleagues[31] used a model-based study to compare effectiveness and cost-effectiveness of EVT versus open revascularization in patients diagnosed with CMI refractory to conservative treatment. Results indicated that EVT is preferred to open revascularization. Even though more interventions are anticipated for patients treated with EVT, this treatment method provides increased quality-adjusted life years and seems to be cost-effective for all ages compared with open vascularization.

NURSING CONSIDERATIONS

A variety of nursing considerations for critically patients are essential in the management of mesenteric ischemia. Supplemental oxygen and infusion of crystalloids should be instituted and maintained as ordered. Vasopressors and anticoagulants, if required, should be infused and monitored. Broad-spectrum antibiotics should be administered as prescribed. The patient's vital signs, urine output, mental status, and peripheral perfusion should be assessed at frequent time intervals to evaluate organ/tissue perfusion. Care should be taken to carefully monitor for fluid overload. Bowel sounds should be auscultated routinely to determine peristaltic activity, and abdominal girth should be measured to assess for distention. Patients should be prepared for endovascular or surgical revascularization as indicated. Observant monitoring for access-related bleeding, such as hematoma, is warranted for patients who have undergone EVT.

Patients should be monitored for sudden and/or unexplained abdominal pain, nausea, vomiting, and diarrhea after any type of invasive procedure. Patients who have undergone cardiac surgery, in particular, should be monitored for the presence of signs that may be associated with development of nonocclusive mesenteric ischemia. Any deterioration in a patient's condition should be reported immediately.

The focus of long-term care for patients who have been diagnosed with and/or treated for mesenteric ischemia is managing risk factors and comorbid conditions. Therefore, patient education should include smoking cessation, dietary changes, and taking any indicated posttreatment medications (eg, blood pressure, antiplatelet, anticoagulant, and/or statin) as directed. The importance of immediately reporting recurrence of symptoms to the health care provider should be emphasized to the patient because of the risk of occlusion or restenosis.

SUMMARY

Mesenteric ischemia is a problematic clinical condition with various causes. Despite advances in diagnostic and management techniques, the early diagnosis and prognosis of AMI remains poor. Long-term survival is limited because of the associated risks and comorbidities. Elderly patients with a delayed diagnosis who subsequently develop peritonitis or organ failure typically have a much worse prognosis. Early diagnosis via CT angiography and prompt revascularization via EVT are recommended for symptomatic patients with AMI or CMI who have not yet developed bowel ischemia and necrosis. Future research on biochemical markers to aid in early diagnosis is needed.

REFERENCES

1. Tilsed JVT, Casamassima A, Kurihara H, et al. ESTES guidelines: acute mesenteric ischaemia. Eur J Trauma Emerg Surg 2016;42(2):253–70.
2. Clair DG, Beach JM. Mesenteric ischemia. N Engl J Med 2016;374(10):959–68.
3. Mastoraki A, Mastoraki S, Tziava E, et al. Mesenteric ischemia: pathogenesis and challenging diagnostic and therapeutic modalities. World J Gastrointest Pathophysiol 2016;7(1):125–30.
4. Carver TW, Vora RS, Taneja A. Mesenteric ischemia. Crit Care Clin 2016;32:155–71.
5. Leone M, Bechis C, Baumstarck K, et al. Outcome of acute mesenteric ischemia in the intensive care unit: a retrospective, multicenter study of 780 cases. Intensive Care Med 2015;41(4):667–76.
6. Bobadilla JL. Mesenteric ischemia. Surg Clin North Am 2013;93(4):925–40.
7. Beaulieu RJ, Arnaoutakis KD, Abularrage CJ, et al. Comparison of open and endovascular treatment of acute mesenteric ischemia. J Vasc Surg 2014;59(1):159–64.
8. Plumereau F, Mucci S, Le Naoures P, et al. Original article: acute mesenteric ischemia of arterial origin: importance of early revascularization. J Visc Surg 2015;152(1):17–22.
9. van den Heijkant TC, Aerts BAC, Teijink JA, et al. Challenges in diagnosing mesenteric ischemia. World J Gastroenterol 2013;19(9):1338–41.
10. Akyildiz HY, Sozuer E, Uzer H, et al. The length of necrosis and renal insufficiency predict the outcome of acute mesenteric ischemia. Asian J Surg 2015;38(1):28–32.

11. Foley TR, Rogers RK. Endovascular therapy for chronic mesenteric ischemia. Curr Treat Options Cardiovasc Med 2016;18(6):1–11.
12. Sise MJ. Acute mesenteric ischemia. Surg Clin North Am 2014;94(1):165–81.
13. AbuRahma AF, Campbell JE, Stone PA, et al. Clinical research study: perioperative and late clinical outcomes of percutaneous transluminal stentings of the celiac and superior mesenteric arteries over the past decade. J Vasc Surg 2013;57: 1052–61.
14. Eris C, Yavuz S, Yalcinkaya S, et al. Acute mesenteric ischemia after cardiac surgery: an analysis of 52 patients. ScientificWorldJournal 2013;2013:631534, e8.
15. Kärkkäinen J, Lehtimäki T, Saari P, et al. Endovascular therapy as a primary revascularization modality in acute mesenteric ischemia. Cardiovasc Intervent Radiol 2015;38(5):1119–29.
16. Yun WS, Lee KK, Cho J, et al. Treatment outcome in patients with acute superior mesenteric artery embolism. Ann Vasc Surg 2013;27(5):613–20.
17. Grilli CJ, Fedele CR, Tahir OM, et al. Clinical study: recanalization of chronic total occlusions of the superior mesenteric artery in patients with chronic mesenteric ischemia: technical and clinical outcomes. J Vasc Interv Radiol 2014;25:1515–22.
18. Acosta S. Mesenteric ischemia. Curr Opin Crit Care 2015;21(2):171–8.
19. Groesdonk HV, Schlempp S, Bomberg H, et al. Risk factors for nonocclusive mesenteric ischemia after elective cardiac surgery. J Thorac Cardiovasc Surg 2013;145(6):1603–10.
20. Cudnik MT, Darbha S, Jones J, et al. The diagnosis of acute mesenteric ischemia: a systematic review and meta-analysis. Acad Emerg Med 2013;20(11):1087–100.
21. Barret M, Martineau C, Rahmi G, et al. Chronic mesenteric ischemia: a rare cause of chronic abdominal pain. Am J Med 2015;128(12):1363.e1–8.
22. Ambe PC, Kang K, Papadakis M, et al. Can the preoperative serum lactate level predict the extent of bowel ischemia in patients presenting to the emergency department with acute mesenteric ischemia? Biomed Res Int 2017;2017: 838795, e5.
23. Branco BC, Aziz H, Montero-Baker MF, et al. Endovascular therapy for acute mesenteric ischemia: an NSQIP analysis. Am Surg 2015;81(11):1170–6.
24. Zhao Y, Yin H, Yao C, et al. Management of acute mesenteric ischemia: a critical review and treatment algorithm. Vasc Endovascular Surg 2016;50(3):183–92.
25. Cai W, Li X, Shu C, et al. Clinical research: comparison of clinical outcomes of endovascular versus open revascularization for chronic mesenteric ischemia: a meta-analysis. Ann Vasc Surg 2015;29:934–40.
26. Björnsson S, Resch T, Acosta S. Symptomatic mesenteric atherosclerotic disease—lessons learned from the diagnostic workup. J Gastrointest Surg 2013; 17:973–80.
27. Oderich GS, Erdoes LS, Lesar C, et al. Comparison of covered stents versus bare metal stents for treatment of chronic atherosclerotic mesenteric arterial disease. J Vasc Surg 2013;58(5):1316–23.
28. Lejay A, Georg Y, Tartaglia E, et al. Chronic mesenteric ischemia: 20 year experience of open surgical treatment. Eur J Vasc Endovasc Surg 2015;49(5):587–92.
29. Moghadamyeghaneh Z, Carmichael JC, Mills SD, et al. Early outcome of treatment of chronic mesenteric ischemia. Am Surg 2015;81(11):1149–56.
30. Li SY, Chen YT, Yang WC, et al. Mesenteric ischemia in patients with end-stage renal disease: a nationwide longitudinal study. Am J Nephrol 2012;35(6):491–7.
31. Hogendoorn W, Hunink MGM, Schlosser FJV, et al. A comparison of open and endovascular revascularization for chronic mesenteric ischemia in a clinical decision model. J Vasc Surg 2014;60(3):715–25.

Clostridium difficile
More Challenging than Ever

Shelley C. Moore, PhD, MSN, RN

KEYWORDS

- *Clostridium difficile* • *C difficile* infection • Fecal microbiota transplant

KEY POINTS

- Although *Clostridium difficile* infection (CDI) is not new and has been present in the hospital environment for more than 30 years, it has now reached epidemic proportions in the United States.
- CDI is classified according to severity: mild, mild-to-moderate, and severe and complicated, with different clinical manifestations and treatment guidelines associated with each classification.
- Evidence points to lack of provider compliance with pharmacologic guidelines.
- Although it is firmly established that antibiotic use is highly linked to CDI, there are other predictive factors of which nurses and physicians should be aware.
- Interdisciplinary collaboration is essential for comprehensive care of patients affected by CDI.

INTRODUCTION

Clostridium difficile is a gram-positive, anaerobic, cytotoxin-producing, spore-forming bacillus that currently rivals all other health care–associated infections, including methicillin-resistant *Staphylococcus aureus*. Although *C difficile* infection (CDI) is not new and has been present in the hospital environment for more than 30 years, it has now reached epidemic proportions[1] and is described by the Centers for Disease Control and Prevention (CDC) as an "urgent threat infection because of its potential to become highly resistant to antibiotics."[2(p1)] CDI is the top cause of health care–associated infectious diarrhea.

PATHOPHYSIOLOGY

Several bacteria live in the gastrointestinal tract (intestinal microbiota). They are important to biologic balance in the gut. These "healthy flora" have a protective role in preventing disease caused by the colonization of pathogens. Administration of

Disclosure: The author has nothing to disclose.
Middle Tennessee State University, School of Nursing, CKNB Box 81, Rm 230, 1301 East Main Street, Murfreesboro, TN 37132, USA
E-mail address: shelley.moore@mtsu.edu

broad-spectrum antibiotics can eliminate these protective flora, which causes the gut to lose its resistance to the *C difficile* bacteria (*C difficile*). Loss of resistance allows *C difficile* spores, which have entered the body via a fecal-oral pathway, to germinate and multiply to high colonization levels and overtake the intestinal niche. The spores form vegetative cells that attach to the epithelial lining of the intestine. Toxins are released, causing infected diarrhea for the individual. The diarrhea occurs because toxins that enter the intestinal wall create increased cell permeability, secretions, and inflammation. *C difficile* spores are strong and durable and thrive in the anaerobic environment of the gut. They are also very hardy in surviving on many inanimate surfaces outside the body for 3 to 6 months. Patients with CDI excrete a large amount of infectious spores in each gram of feces. Feces can get on health care workers' (and patients') hands and other objects in the environment, such as bedside tables, side rails, door knobs, even computer equipment, and be passed from person to person or object to person. Because the spores can remain in a dormant state so long, everyone in the setting is at risk, including health care workers, and especially vulnerable patients who can serve as an unsuspecting host for these spores.[1,3] The cycle continues.

DIAGNOSIS

CDI is diagnosed by laboratory and radiographic studies as well as clinical symptoms and history. Different facilities perform different tests on the patient's diarrhea stool; whatever specific methods a laboratory uses typically includes cultures, tests for toxins, and measures polymerase chain reactions (PCR). Formed stool should never be used as a specimen because it can generate false positives.[3] Practice guidelines supported with strong evidence and published in the American Journal of Gastroenterology (2013) state that (1) nucleic acid amplification tests (NAAT) for *C difficile* toxin genes such as PCR are superior to toxins A + B E1A testing; and (2) glutamate dehydrogenase screening tests for *C difficile* can be used in 2- or 3-step screening algorithms with subsequent toxin A + B E1A testing, but the sensitivity of this is lower than NAATs. These guidelines concede that the best standard laboratory test has not yet been confirmed, but that *C difficile* culture alone is not adequate because not all strains emit toxins.[4(pp479,480)]

Abdominal CT scan is a useful diagnostic tool. Changes in the colonic wall can be detected. Advantages of CT are as follows: the relative accuracy, noninvasiveness, quickness, and the ability to monitor serially. Repeat stool testing is not recommended. Laboratory methods continue to be studied, and it is hoped improved upon. Endoscopy is not recommended because of its cost and risks.[5]

CLINICAL MANIFESTATIONS

C difficile causes intestinal inflammation. CDI is defined as "acute onset of diarrhea with documented toxigenic *C difficile* or its toxin and no other documented cause for diarrhea."[4] The clinical manifestations can range from asymptomatic carrier or mild self-resolving diarrhea to copious diarrhea with resulting pseudomembranous colitis, sepsis, and death.[6] CDI is classified according to severity: mild, mild-to-moderate, and severe and complicated. Symptoms can manifest shortly after antibiotic therapy or not until months later. Mild CDI exhibits as diarrhea only. Mild-to-moderate CDI exhibits diarrhea plus fever, chills, dehydration, poor skin turgor, dry mucous membranes, nausea, and anorexia. There is foul-smelling and/or bloody diarrhea, abdominal distention, and abdominal pain ranging from minor cramping to pronounced and diffuse pain. With severe and complicated CDI, pseudomembranous colitis (severe acute inflammation of the bowel mucosa with the formation of mucinous exudate patches) may be present, and laboratory values are abnormal. Serum albumin is <3 d/dL, plus *one* of the following: hypotension with or without use of vasopressors, white blood cell (WBC) count greater than 15,000/μL, abdominal tenderness, serum lactate levels greater than 2.2 mmol/L, profuse diarrhea, pain in lower part of abdomen, leukocytosis, severe abdominal pain, high fever (>38.5°C or 101.3°F), chills, abdominal distention. These patients need to be admitted to the intensive care unit (ICU) or may already be there. If the patient has an ileus, they may have minimal diarrhea. The patient can have severe CDI and not have pseudomembranous colitis. If the patient does have pseudomembranous colitis (sometimes called fulminant colitis), complications may include toxic megacolon (acute, life-threatening dilation of the colon), perforation of the colon, and death. There is a fourth category of CDI, which is recurrent CDI (RCDI), defined as CDI recurring within 8 weeks of completion of therapy.[3] RCDI is especially hard to treat.

PREVALENCE AND COST BURDEN

In 2011, CDI was reported to be responsible for 453,000 infections and 29,000 deaths.[7] Estimates are that the diagnosis and treatment of CDI cost more than $3.2 billion per year in the United States. CDI is among the most common health care–associated infections in both hospitalized patients and residents of long-term care facilities. The incidence of severe and RCDI has increased because of new strains of *C difficile* resistant to traditional medications.[3]

Dubberke and Olsen[8(pS88)] state that the "total burden of CDI on the healthcare system is significantly underestimated." This statement makes sense because almost all studies in the literature are based on CDIs diagnosed and managed in the hospital setting. CDI is becoming more prominent in the long-term care setting and in the community, thus "the focus of published studies solely on inpatient hospital diagnosis and treatment of CDI ignores the contribution of other healthcare costs to the economic burden of CDI."[8(pS88)] Recent research is just beginning to include associations with long-term care facilities and is discussed later.

According to the CDC, methicillin-resistant *S aureus* cases are decreasing, whereas CDI cases are increasingly rapidly.[1] During the last decade, CDI incidence has risen in developed countries. Increased incidence causes great concern. Bouza and colleagues[9(p543)] identify this as a "potential marker of deficiencies in antimicrobial stewardship."

RISK FACTORS AND PREDICTORS

What is "antibiotic stewardship" and why is it important? Antimicrobial stewardship programs are often connected with treatment (and prevention) of CDI. There are several components to antibiotic/antimicrobial stewardship. Two of them specific to providers are the following: (1) ensuring that patients are receiving optimal care for their infections; and (2) guideline development and adherence to these via "order sets."[7] Additional aspects of good stewardship include the following: (1) providers prescribing antibiotics only for bacterial infections and not viruses; (2) avoiding overuse/abuse of antibiotics; (3) patient taking the antibiotic exactly as prescribed; (4) patients taking only their own prescription and not someone else's; and (5) prescribing narrow-based antibiotic sensitive to a certain organism versus use of broad-spectrum antibiotic that will kill off normal, protective flora. The antibiotic culprits most guilty of contributing to opportunistic development of *C difficile* are as follows: clindamycin, cephalosporins, penicillins, and fluoroquinolones. Sometimes even one dose of an antibiotic can precipitate CDI.[1] A perfect setup for this to happen would be a patient in an outpatient (or inpatient) surgical setting getting a surgical procedure whereby the protocol is to give a dose of antibiotic immediately before skin incision as a measure to prevent surgical site infection. Depending upon the patient's health status and comorbidities, this can be enough to tip the scale toward a CDI. There are plenty of dormant *C difficile* spores clinging to surfaces in the setting and hands of health care workers, waiting for a susceptible host to ingest them.

Although it is firmly established that antibiotic use is highly linked to CDI, there are other predictive factors. Several studies have investigated risk factors, and some have tried to create predictive models. Age is definitely an independent predictor. More than 90% of annual deaths caused by *C difficile* happen in people greater than the age of 65 years. Some evidence indicates that "the percentage of CDI patients with severe outcomes increased with each decade of age beginning at age 60."[10(p1219)] A study by Chopra and colleagues[10] investigated the independent predictors of death within 30 days of CDI diagnosis among patients $\geq$ age 60 who were admitted to a tertiary care hospital in Detroit. A matched cases-to-control design was used. Their study illuminated the independent predictor, serum creatinine (SrCr). This finding was aligned with other similar studies. "An elevated SrCr level may signify a severe course of disease because it is indicative of severe diarrhea or sepsis caused by CDI, resulting in inadequate renal perfusion."[10(p1222)]

Of interest is that this study did not result in the same predictors as other studies the samples of which were CDI cases in the general population (not restricted by age $\geq$60). Predictors in the general population were elevated WBC count, low albumin, and high body temperature. Older adults do not always exhibit the same signs and symptoms of infection as younger adults, for example leukocytosis and fever. Many older adults often run a low albumin level to begin with, often as a result of changed nutrition. Older adults in any setting, but especially in long-term care settings and hospitals, need heightened vigilance for preventing CDI.[10]

Often associated with advanced age is poor functional status. In an investigation exploring the relationship between functional status and CDI severity, Rao and colleagues[11] found that the activities of daily living classification, full assistance, and the mental health condition, depression, were strongly positively correlated with severe CDI. A strength of this study was that it was prospective, whereas most studies on CDI in the literature are retrospective.

Patients 65 and older with poor functional status are often seen in the ICU. A common syndrome is that of delirium, which occurs even more frequently in elderly patients. A study by Archbald-Pannone and colleagues[6] concluded that patients who were diagnosed in the ICU and developed delirium are at the highest risk for dying within 30 days of CDI diagnosis. In their model, they included the Charlson comorbidity index, WBC, blood urea nitrogen, ICU location at diagnosis, location admitted from, and delirium, and then used logistic regression statistics on the 362-patient sample. Albumin level was not included in the model because they collected this value on only 87% of the sample. In following the study patients for 30 days, they found that delirium was the strongest predictor of death after CDI, followed by admission from long-term care. Discovering this strong relationship with delirium is important because "delirium is under-recognized, underdiagnosed, and underreported in hospitalized patients."[6(p691)] Because it can be reversed, it is extremely important to identify delirium early on. Identification of delirium is facilitated by using an assessment tool such as the Confusion Assessment Method.[6]

Many studies, including the ones described above, have either suggested the development of or tried to create, a bedside assessment tool to assess risk factors for CDI in order to better care for patients. Some researchers have gone so far as to both develop an assessment tool and then actually implement it. Although this is a very aggressive research methodology, valuable information can come from this type of study. One such study is that of Cruz-Betancourt and colleagues.[12] Using their predictive screening tool, they then implemented a "bundle of mitigation interventions."[12(p421)] The study was done in a vascular-thoracic intensive care unit (VTICU) with high rates of hospital-acquired CDI. The 3 most common risk factors they found in their patient population were use of a proton-pump inhibitor or H_2 antagonist, the concurrent use of multiple antibiotic agents, and mechanical ventilation. As ICU nurses know, these factors are frequently present in ICU patients. They also looked at other variables, such as age, gender, length of stay in both the hospital and the VTICU, days on antibiotics, history of immunosuppression, gastrointestinal procedures or surgery, dialysis, whether admitted from long-term care or another hospital, serum albumin, enteral feedings, laxatives, and steroids. Based on the data results, they came up with the following preventive measures (**Table 1**). Implementation of these interventions yielded a decrease in the VTICU's CDI rate. Neither the screening tool devised nor the interventions can be generalized to all hospital ICUs, but it worked for this one. Another limitation is that, because these are "bundles," it is impossible to know which, if any, of the interventions made the most difference. The researchers recommended further study related to more proactive identification of at-risk patients and prevention measures in other settings.

Davis and colleagues[2] also implemented "bundles" and studied effectiveness on CDI. **Table 2** describes these bundles. This study was also single centered. Their bundle approach focused on multidisciplinary efforts, as did the Cruz-Betancourt study.[2,12] The Davis study was published as a "Brief Report" in *American Journal of Infection Control*, so there was not a great deal of information on the methods and data results; however, there was a significant reduction in CDI in the group that experienced the preventative bundles.

Table 1
Preventive measures applied during the Cruz-Betancourt and colleagues study (2016)

Intervention Category (ie, Bundle)	Description of Intervention
Identification	Identification of patients at high risk by placing magnet on doorframe
Infection preventionist	• Notifies Infection Prevention Department, ESD, and unit-based nurse leadership of patients at high risk • Notifies bedside nurse of patients at high risk and provides 1:1 education on infection prevention strategies • Places bleach disposable wipes outside and inside patient rooms • Patient education regarding infection prevention
Pharmacologic	• Proton pump inhibitors changed to an H_2 antagonist • Discontinuation of acid suppression therapy • Discontinuation of laxatives • Discontinuation of steroids • Add probiotics • Discontinuation or adjustment of antibiotic agents
Environmental Services Department (ESD)	• ESD consistently cleans high-touch areas using chlorine agent

Adapted from Cruz-Betancourt A, Cooper CD, Sposato K, et al. Effects of a predictive preventive model for prevention of Clostridium difficile infection in patients in intensive care units. Am J Infect Control 2016;44(4):423; with permission.

Table 2
Bundles for prevention of *Clostridium difficile* infection

Bundle Intervention	Description
Antimicrobial and drug management	• Evidence-based management and treatment • Judicious use of all antibiotics • Robust antibiotic stewardship program led by Pharmacy and physician champion • Assess use of probiotics • Assess use of proton pump inhibitors • Educate providers and patients
Detection	• Early recognition: simple diagnosis • Testing criteria • Proper collection and handling of specimens (timeframe and temperature) • Appropriate testing: PCR, antigen/toxin assay • Retesting criteria: no testing for cure
Cleaning	• Environment • Equipment: identify *C diff*–contaminated equipment for cleaning • Daily cleaning • Terminal cleaning • Use of checklist • Appropriate dwell time for cleaning solutions • Competency assessment
Practice	• Early isolation • Contact precautions: gowns, gloves, signage, hand hygiene with soap and water (NOT hand sanitizer) • Equipment: available, dedicated, disposable, disinfected if reusable
People	• Administrative support • Competency • Compliance • Coach • Communicative • Involve and educate patients/families • Educate all staff • Collaborative efforts beyond the hospital

Adapted from Davis BM, Yin J, Blomberg D, et al. Impact of a prevention bundle on Clostridium difficile infection rates in a hospital in the southeastern United States. Am J Infect Control 2016;44:1730; with permission.

Other studies have focused on the particular strain of the *C difficile* bacteria. Most mentioned in the literature is the ribotype 027 strain. One study found that patients infected with the 027 strain had higher mortalities and more inflammation than non-027 strains. There was also a significant positive correlation between patients from long-term care settings and the 027 strain.[13] Strain 027 has certain characteristics that may cause increased severity of CDI. 027 is thought to have increased toxin production, higher levels of colonization, and higher risk for recurrence. The use of fluoroquinolones in addition to age greater than 65 is now associated with highest risk for the 027 strain.[1] The 027 strain is thought to be directly associated with higher mortality due to fulminant colitis.[5] Although 027 is the current epidemic strain, it is expected that new strains will surface. There are preliminary reports of ribotype 078 coming onto the scene in Europe, where the prevalence of the 027 strain has decreased.[1]

TREATMENT

Way back in 1995, the Society for Healthcare Epidemiology of America (SHEA) disseminated a clinical position paper declaring metronidazole and vancomycin equally effective, but mentioned that metronidazole may be preferred to avoid vancomycin resistance. Fifteen years later, SHEA along with the Infectious Diseases Society of America (IDSA) published new guidelines. The new guidelines were devised in response to increased prevalence, severity, and drug resistance of CDI. The new guidelines recommended vancomycin as the first-line drug for the classification of severe CDI while keeping the recommendation of metronidazole for mild-moderate.[14] In 2013, the American College of Gastroenterology concurred with the SHEA/IDSA guidelines.[15] An important question is: are providers actually following these guidelines? At least 2 studies have explored this.

Curtin[14] assessed a tertiary care academic medical center's compliance with the SHEA/IDSA guidelines and found overall compliance to be poor, particularly with regard to severe disease. Full adherence to the guidelines was found in 65.9% of the mild-moderate cases, only 25.3% in severe cases, and only 35.5% of the complicated cases, for an overall mean of 65.9%. This study showed that physicians correctly treated mild-moderate cases with metronidazole (perhaps because this was the original 1995 recommendation), but that then they unfortunately also treated severe and complicated cases with metronidazole, wherein they should have used vancomycin. The study also revealed only partial compliance with the guidelines in that often the correct drug was chosen for the degree of severity, but the wrong dosage was chosen. In addition to physician education on the 2010 guidelines and antibiotic stewardship, the investigators suggest that the guidelines should be updated to specifically address the pharmacologic management of CDI patients who also have renal disease and are immunosuppressed.

Brown and Seifert[15] conducted a similar study, and found similar results, at another tertiary care referral county teaching hospital. Concern over increased severity, disease prevalence, especially of the highly virulent strain ribotype 027 (also known as North American Pulsed Field type I [NAP-1]), and resistance to standard therapy drove their study. This study was different from Curtin[14] in that it looked at outcomes. The aim was to determine if compliance with the drug treatment guidelines lowered rates of CDI complications. Complications were defined as follows: infection recurrence; any surgical intervention intended to cure the CDI; a diagnosis of toxic megacolon; and mortality within 30 days. Like the Curtin study, Brown and Seifert's results showed that guideline-compliant treatment was more likely to be administered in mild-moderate CDI than in severe or complicated CDI (81.2% vs 35.3% and 19.7%, respectively). As CDI complexity increased, compliance with guidelines (guideline-concordance) decreased. As guideline-concordance decreased, RCDI (recurrence) increased. The most common reasons for discordance with guidelines for treatment of mild-moderate CDI were as follows: (1) treating a multiple recurrence with metronidazole instead of vancomycin; and (2) failing to use a tapered ("pulsed") regimen to prevent additional recurrences. The most common reasons for discordance with guidelines for treatment of severe and complicated CDI were as follows: (1) treating with metronidazole instead of vancomycin; and (2) failing to use a tapered regimen. The more noncompliant or discordant with guidelines, the more complications.[15]

Both of the above studies reflect that quality of care is lacking. Furthermore, Brown and Seifert point out that "it has been estimated that American patients receive only slightly more than half of recommended care during health care visits."[15(p869)] They meant health care visits in general, not just for CDI, and also noted that, in their study, "most patients were treated initially by residents from both Family and Internal Medicine teams. Infectious Disease specialists were rarely involved, which could account for the low rates of guideline-concordant therapy."[15(p870)] Perhaps Infectious Disease specialists would have been more familiar with the guidelines. **Tables 3** and **4** provide the SHEA/IDSA guidelines. Because these guidelines are now several years old, modifications should be made. The authors of the guidelines say as much by stating, "the initial step in developing a rational clinical research agenda is the identification of gaps in information," and they concede that there are gaps in their 2010 guidelines. They recommend further research and refinement, including that for treatment guidelines.[16(pp448,449)] Two of the many treatment questions they pose are as follows: if a valid severity-of-illness tool for CDI is developed, how will treatment recommendations for both primary and recurrent CDI change? What is the best approach to treatment of fulminant CDI?[16]

Three years after the SHEA/IDSA guidelines were published, Surawicz and colleagues[4] proposed drug guidelines not significantly different than SHEA/IDSA, but there are some subtle modifications. Also, their criteria are different, and they add a comment about suggested alternative treatments. A 2016 study by Akamine and colleagues[17] indicated that, even though patients who had received intracolonic vancomycin were sicker (thus the need for intracolonic route), they had a similar mortality to the group who received standard route therapy. As this was a retrospective study, prospective randomized controlled trials are needed in this area to assess the efficacy of this potentially valuable adjunctive treatment.

A systematic review by Stewart and colleagues[18] concluded that there is a small survival benefit for fulminant colitis patients who undergo a colectomy with end ileostomy versus those who continue to receive standard medical therapy. Fulminant colitis is thought to occur in only 2% to 5% of CDI patients but has a mortality of 35% to 80%. Usually it is accompanied by severe abdominal pain and distention, worsening

Table 3
C difficile treatment recommendations from Society for Healthcare Epidemiology of America/Infectious Diseases Society of America

Clinical Definition	Criteria	Recommended Treatment
Initial episode, mild or moderate	Leukocytosis with a WBC ≥15,000 and SrCr <1.5 times baseline level	Metronidazole, 500 mg, 3 times per day PO for 10–14 d
Initial episode, severe	Leukocytosis with a WBC ≥15,000 OR an SrCr ≥1.5 times baseline	Vancomycin, 125 mg, 4 times per day PO for 10–14 d
Initial episode, severe, complicated	Hypotension or shock, ileus, megacolon	Vancomycin, 500 mg, 4 times PO or by nasogastric tube, plus metronidazole 500 mg every 8 h intravenously. If complete ileus, consider adding rectal instillation of vancomycin
First recurrence	—	Same as for initial episode
Second recurrence	—	Vancomycin in a tapered or pulsed regimen

Adapted from Brown AT, Seifert CF. Effect of treatment variation on outcomes in patients with Clostridium difficile. Am J Med 2014;127(9):876, with permission; and Cohen SH, Gerding DN, Johnson S, et al. Clinical practice guidelines for Clostridium difficile infection in adults: 2010 update by the Society for Healthcare Epidemiology of America (SHEA) and the Infectious Diseases Society of America (IDSA). Infect Control Hosp Epidemiol 2010;31(5):447; with permission.

Table 4
Clostridium difficile infection severity scoring system and summary of recommended treatments

Severity	Criteria	Treatment	Comment
Mild-moderate diagnosis	Diarrhea plus any additional signs or symptoms not meeting server or complicated criteria	Metronidazole, 500 mg, 3 times per day PO for 10 d. If unable to take metronidazole, vancomycin 125 mg PO 4 times per day for 10 d	If no improvement in 5–7 d, consider change to vancomycin at standard dose (12 mg 4 times per day)
Severe disease	Serum albumin <3 g/dL plus ONE of the following: WBC ≥15,000 Abdominal tenderness	Vancomycin 125 mg PO 4 times per day for 10 d	—
Severe and complicated disease	Any of the following attributable to CDI: • Admission to ICU for CDI • Hypotension with/without use of vasopressors • Fever ≥38.5°C • Ileus or significant abdominal distension • Mental status changes • WBC ≥35,000 or <2 cells/mm³ • Serum lactate levels >2.2 mmol/L • End-organ failure (mechanical ventilation, renal failure, and so forth)	Vancomycin 500 mg PO 4 times per day and metronidazole 500 mg IV every 8 h, and vancomycin per rectum (vancomycin 500 mg in 500 mL saline as enema) 4 times per day	Surgical consultation
Recurrent CDI	Recurrent CDI within 8 wk of completion of therapy	Repeat metronidazole or vancomycin pulse regimen	Consider FMT after 3 recurrences

Adapted from Surawicz CM, Brandt LJ, Binion DG, et al. Guidelines for diagnosis, treatment, and prevention of Clostridium difficile infections. Am J Gastroenterol 2013;108(4):482; with permission.

diarrhea, and often hypotension, altered mental status, and end-organ failure. The patient can be septic, intubated, and in renal failure. A lack of diarrhea with worsening abdominal distention is an "ominous finding and is indicative of ileus and intestinal failure"—something critical care nurses should be aware of.[5(p26)] The total colectomy with end ileostomy is a very high-risk surgery in a critically ill patient. An alternative surgical strategy that is less invasive and done earlier could possibly improve postoperative mortalities. "One emerging option is laparoscopic creation of a double-barrel ileostomy for distal colonic washout….The surgical intervention involve(s) the creation of a loop ileostomy, intraoperative colonic lavage with warmed polyethylene glycol 3350/electrolyte solution via the ileostomy, and postoperative antegrade instillation of vancomycin flushes via the ileostomy….Long-term outcomes and risk of recurrence remain to be assessed."[5(p31)]

Because the prevalence of recurrent or refractory CDI is on the increase, nonsurgical alternatives need to be considered. Perhaps the most promising choice, but not very popular yet, is fecal microbiota transplant (FMT). It is inexpensive, safe, and efficient. The American College of Gastroenterology "recommends FMT after a third RCDI in order to reestablish the normal composition of the gut flora, restore the balance in metabolism, and stimulate both cellular and humoral immune responses in the gut mucosa."[3(p56)] In FMT, the stool of a healthy donor is mixed with saline or water, filtered to remove larger particles, and then instilled into the gastrointestinal tract of an RCDI patient. The most common method of administration used to be retention enema, but newer methods include nasogastric tube, nasoduodenal tube, colonoscopy, and oral fecal capsules. Nasogastric tube administration is the easiest and has a 73% to 83% success rate. The colonoscopy method is advantageous because (1) the substance can be infused throughout the length of the colon; (2) the colon mucosa can be directly observed for abnormalities; (3) it is tolerated well by the patient; and (4) success rate for cure is 86% to 100%. Risks present with this method are perforation, infection, bleeding, and pain. Donors need to be screened for CDI.[3]

IMPLICATIONS FOR NURSES

Nurses play a major role in prevention of, identification for risk of, and management of, CDI.

Prevention begins with meticulous hand washing with soap and running water, NOT hand sanitizer. It is necessary to mechanically remove spores from hands and decrease cross-contamination. Alcohol-based sanitizer merely causes redistribution of the spores over the hands and wrists. Nurses must involve patients and families/visitors in proper hand hygiene, including hand to mouth warning. Use of appropriate personal protective equipment, conscientious environmental cleaning, use of disposable equipment, patient advocacy and antibiotic stewardship, careful monitoring of laboratory values and patient signs/symptoms, correct specimen collection, and facilitation of interdisciplinary collaboration are essential nursing responsibilities. Safe and supportive care for CDI patients is crucial because these are some of the sickest patients for whom a nurse can be charged with caring.[3,5] An extremely good tip for critical care nurses is that collaboration with "hospitalists and gastroenterologists to provide the most current treatment options" is required.

FUTURE RESEARCH

FMT has shown great promise as a very efficacious treatment, but it needs more randomized controlled clinical trials. Nursing researchers can contribute by studying patient understanding and acceptance, and clinical management and outcomes for FMT versus traditional treatments. With more and more incidence of RCDI, FMT will receive more accolades. FMT has the potential to increase patients' resistance to CDI and even reduce other inflammatory diseases, such as inflammatory bowel disease, irritable bowel syndrome, obesity, Parkinson disease, anxiety, and autism; however, far more research is needed.[3(pp60–62)] Reflection on these conditions is beyond the scope of this article but warrants further inspection.

Although ribotype 027 (also known as NAP1) is the current epidemic strain, other strains are on the horizon (for example, 078). Because the host immune response plays such an important role in CDI, vaccines need to be studied (and are). The thought is to possibly vaccinate target populations, such as elective surgery patients who get admitted, at-risk older adults facing admission to long-term care, and people with chronic conditions that are associated with frequent hospital admissions (chronic obstructive pulmonary disease, diabetes, renal failure). A feasible vaccine has not yet been approved.[1]

New antibiotics also need to be developed. The newest one is Fidaxomicin (2011), marketed as Dificid by Optimer Pharmaceuticals, and was the first new drug to be approved specifically for CDI in 25 years. Fidaxomicin is a narrow spectrum macrocylic and somewhat spares the normal intestinal flora. Unfortunately, it is very expensive at $3000 for a 10-day course.[1]

Further research is also needed on the role of probiotics in both treating and preventing CDI. Use of probiotics in the critically ill patient is debatable because of the potential risk of bloodstream infection. The current state-of-the-science regarding probiotics is beyond the scope of this article but is a highly relevant topic.[1] Another vast area of intrigue is the increase of seemingly "community-acquired" CDI in populations thought to be at low risk, including children.[1] Even increased understanding of disinfectants is a research need. Although chlorine-releasing agents are thought to be the most effective in killing spores, it is uncertain whether this actually leads to decreased incidence of CDI.[1]

SUMMARY

CDI is a serious public health threat. In 2010, members of the SHEA-IDSA Expert Panel and of the IDSA Research Committee outlined a research agenda that has not been thoroughly vetted as of yet. They identified key clinical areas to focus upon.

Epidemiology

Little is known about the incubation period of *C difficile* and its infectious dose. More understanding is needed concerning administration of proton pump inhibitors and risk of CDI.[16]

With so many people taking proton pump inhibitors, information on this is crucial. The role of asymptomatic carriers in transmission, especially in the health care setting, is another mystery.[16]

Diagnostics

There is a variety of tests used to detect *C difficile*. There are many unanswered questions on which are the most sensitive, which method is best when a hospital does not have PCR technology, and whether repeat stool testing can be valuable.[16] The lack of standardization here adversely affects quality of care.

Prevention

What preventive measures above and beyond hand hygiene, environmental management, and antibiotic stewardship can be taken against CDI? The right combination of probiotics, an effective and timely vaccine, and serologic biomarkers to appropriately assess immunity and predict CDI[16] would all be more proactive than what is available now.

Nursing Diagnosis and Management

Until standard assessment tools for CDI can be validated and implemented, the bedside nurse's physical assessment skills are all the more important. Nurses should obtain a thorough history from patients who have diarrhea. They should ascertain antibiotic use, recent hospitalization or stay in a nursing home, onset of signs and symptoms, and "whether or not the diarrhea is the primary sign or if a causative agent of the diarrhea has been identified."[3(p59)] Additional things to assess in patients are whether the patient is immunosuppressed, is elderly, or has a history of gastrointestinal disorders.[3] Renal status is another factor to consider. "Holistic assessment of all systems is also important to rapidly detect systemic manifestations"[3(p60)] because presence of CDI may be accompanied by significant illness and comorbidities.

Last but not least, the patient's comfort is a priority. Frequent loose stools, abdominal pain, and risk for skin breakdown are patient concerns for nurses caring for CDI victims.[3] Interdisciplinary collaboration is essential for comprehensive care of patients affected by the rising epidemic of CDI. A particularly vulnerable population of people is those 65 years of age and older.

REFERENCES

1. Ghose C. Clostridium difficile infection in the twenty-first century. Emerg Microbes Infect 2013;2(9):1–8.
2. Davis BM, Yin J, Blomberg D, et al. Impact of a prevention bundle on Clostridium difficile infection rates in a hospital in the southeastern United States. Am J Infect Control 2016;44:1729–31.
3. Boyle ML, Ruth-Sahd LA, Zhou Z. Fecal microbiota transplant to treat recurrent Clostridium difficile infections. Crit Care Nurse 2015;35(2):51–64.
4. Surawicz CM, Brandt LJ, Binion DG, et al. Guidelines for diagnosis, treatment, and prevention of Clostridium difficile infections. Am J Gastroenterol 2013; 108(4):478–98.
5. Walters PR, Zuckerbraun BS. Clostridium difficile infection: clinical challenges and management strategies. Crit Care Nurse 2014;34(4):24–33.
6. Archbald-Pannone LR, McMurry TL, Guerrant RL, et al. Delirium and other clinical factors with Clostridium difficile infection that predict mortality in hospitalized patients. Am J Infect Control 2015;43(7):690–3.
7. Revolinski S. Implementation of a clinical decision support alert for the management of Clostridium difficile infection. Antibiotics (Basel) 2015;4(4): 667–74.
8. Dubberke ER, Olsen MA. Burden of Clostridium difficile on the healthcare system. Clin Infect Dis 2012;55(suppl 2):S88–92.
9. Bouza E, Rodríguez-Créixems M, Alcalá L, et al. Is Clostridium difficile infection an increasingly common severe disease in adult intensive care units? A 10-year experience. J Crit Care 2015;30(3):543–9.
10. Chopra T, Awali RA, Biedron C, et al. Predictors of Clostridium difficile infection–related mortality among older adults. Am J Infect Control 2016;44(11):1219–23.
11. Rao K, Micic D, Chenoweth E, et al. Poor functional status as a risk factor for severe Clostridium difficile infection in hospitalized older adults. J Am Geriatr Soc 2013;61(10):1738–42.
12. Cruz-Betancourt A, Cooper CD, Sposato K, et al. Effects of a predictive preventive model for prevention of Clostridium difficile infection in patients in intensive care units. Am J Infect Control 2016;44(4):421–4.
13. Archbald-Pannone LR, Boone JH, Carman RJ, et al. Clostridium difficile ribotype 027 is most prevalent among inpatients admitted from long-term care facilities. J Hosp Infect 2014;88(4):218–21.
14. Curtin BF. Clostridium difficile -associated disease: adherence with current guidelines at a tertiary medical center. World J Gastroenterol 2013;19(46):8647.
15. Brown AT, Seifert CF. Effect of treatment variation on outcomes in patients with Clostridium difficile. Am J Med 2014;127(9):865–70.

16. Cohen SH, Gerding DN, Johnson S, et al. Clinical practice guidelines for Clostridium difficile infection in adults: 2010 update by the Society for Healthcare Epidemiology of America (SHEA) and the Infectious Diseases Society of America (IDSA). Infect Control Hosp Epidemiol 2010;31(5):431–55.
17. Akamine CM, Ing MB, Jackson CS, et al. The efficacy of intracolonic vancomycin for severe Clostridium difficile colitis: a case series. BMC Infect Dis 2016;16(1): 1–7.
18. Stewart DB, Hollenbeak CS, Wilson MZ. Is colectomy for fulminant Clostridium difficile colitis life saving? A systematic review. Colorectal Dis 2013;15(7): 798–804.

Management of Acute Gastrointestinal Bleed

Francisca Cisneros Farrar, EdD, MSN, RN

KEYWORDS

- Acute gastrointestinal bleeding • Ulcerative erosions
- Complications of portal hypertension • Vascular lesions • Angiodysplasia • Colitis
- Inflammatory bowel disease • Colon cancer

KEY POINTS

- Acute gastrointestinal bleeding is a common problem found in critically ill patients that can range from a self-limited bleeding disorder to a life-threatening hemorrhaging emergency.
- Acute gastrointestinal bleeding is unstable and can quickly become a medical emergency.
- Frontline critical nurses must acquire self-efficacy for management of acute gastrointestinal bleeding disorders.
- The nurse must have knowledge about these disorders and potential complications to develop clinical reasoning skills to identify a change of condition to hemodynamic instability.

INTRODUCTION

Acute gastrointestinal bleeding is a common problem found in critically ill patients that can range from a self-limited bleeding disorder to a life-threatening hemorrhaging emergency. The frontline critical care nurse encounters these common gastrointestinal bleeding disorders in practice settings. Therefore, it is essential that the frontline critical care nurse develop self-efficacy for management of acute gastrointestinal bleeding disorders. The nurse must have knowledge about these disorders and potential complications, and must develop clinical reasoning skills to be able to identify patient changes of condition to hemodynamic instability. The purpose of this article is to overview upper and lower acute gastrointestinal bleeding and provide current evidence-based standards of care for nursing management of acute gastrointestinal bleeding. Common bleeding disorders are reviewed with expanded focus on peptic ulcer, acute variceal hemorrhage, colonic diverticular bleeding, and angiodysplasias, which are commonly found in the critical care setting.

Disclosures: There are no disclosures or conflict of interest for any relationship with a commercial company that has a direct financial interest in subject matter or materials discussed in this article or with a company making a competing product.
Austin Peay State University, School of Nursing, PO Box 4658, Clarksville, TN 37043, USA
E-mail address: farrarf@apsu.edu

ACUTE GASTROINTESTINAL BLEEDING
Pathogenesis

The gastrointestinal tract transports, digests, and eliminates ingested material. A healthy gastrointestinal track supplies nutrients, vitamins, electrolytes, and minerals to the body that are essential to maintaining hemodynamic stability.[1] The gastrointestinal tract also contains clusters of immune cells embedded in the gastrointestinal track to provide immunosurveillance.[1] Injuries to the structure or function results in clinical manifestations that can lead to bleeding disorders and hemodynamic instability.

Gastrointestinal hemorrhage from the upper gastrointestinal track occurs proximal to the ligament of Treitz, whereas lower gastrointestinal tract bleeding occurs distal to the gastrointestinal tract.[2,3] Gastrointestinal bleeding is characterized as upper gastrointestinal when bleeding is from the esophagus, stomach, or duodenum. Gastrointestinal bleeding is characterized as lower gastrointestinal when bleeding is from the jejunum, ileum, or colon.[1,3] The anatomic division of the duodenum and the jejunum by the Treitz ligament division separates the upper and lower gastrointestinal tract, thereby classifying the bleeding as upper or lower.[1-3]

Bleeding Presentation

Clinical presentation of gastrointestinal bleeding includes

- Hematemesis: Vomiting of red or coffee brown appearance
- Melena: Passage of black, tarry stools
- Occult-blood in stool: Not visible to the naked eye; detected by performing a laboratory test on a stool specimen
- Hematochezia: Passage of fresh blood per anus in stools.[2,3]

Common Disorders Associated with Acute Gastrointestinal Bleeding

Gastrointestinal bleeding is a common emergency ranging from acute hemorrhage, triggering the need for resuscitation of the patient with immediate management of hypovolemia, to acute bleeding that stops spontaneously.[3] The frontline nurse needs to be alert to patient change in condition, such as sudden hemorrhage or rebleed that is life-threatening, requiring a medical emergency response. The frontline nurse needs to acquire self-efficacy clinical skills in managing acute gastrointestinal bleeding. Early intervention by the frontline nurse can prevent serious complications, including death.

Common upper gastrointestinal bleeding disorders

Acute upper gastrointestinal bleeding is from the esophagus, stomach, or duodenum. Upper gastrointestinal bleeding can be classified by the anatomic and pathophysiologic factors that lead to a bleeding disorder. These 3 pathogenic causes are ulcerative erosive lesions, complications of portal hypertension, and vascular lesions.[1-3] Common causes of acute upper gastrointestinal bleeding include

- Peptic ulcer: The most common cause for upper gastrointestinal bleeding, it is associated with acute bleeding due to anatomic position to major arteries. This erosive disorder is associated with *Helicobacter pylori* infection, stress, aspirin, and nonsteroidal antiinflammatory drugs (NSAIDs).[3-5]
- Esophageal varices: This disorder is associated with portal hypertension due to liver disease. Causative factors of liver disease include excessive alcohol and hepatitis.[3]
- Malignancy: A common cause is adenocarcinoma of the stomach and gastric lymphoma. Bleeding occurs with ulceration of the mucosal surface.[3]

- Mallory-Weiss tears: Profuse vomiting causes mucosal lesions, followed by hematemesis.[2,3]

Common lower gastrointestinal bleeding disorders

Acute lower gastrointestinal bleeding is from the jejunum, ileum, or colon. This results in hemodynamic instability, anemia, and the possible need for blood transfusions.[1,3] Lower gastrointestinal bleeding can be classified by the 4 anatomic and pathophysiologic factors leading to acute bleeding. These 4 pathogenic causes are anatomic, vascular, inflammatory, and neoplastic factors.[2-4] Causes of lower gastrointestinal bleeding include

- Diverticular disease: Bleeding is common in acute colonic diverticular bleeding. Most bleeds stop spontaneously. After 2 major bleeds, operative intervention should be considered.[2,3]
- Inflammatory bowel disease: Bloody diarrhea is common. Crohn disorder is a risk factor for profuse hemorrhage and rebleed due to inflammatory colitis involving the entire thickness of the bowel. Urgent surgery is usually recommended. Ulcerative colitis presents as bloody diarrhea and ischemic colitis presents as bloody diarrhea accompanied by pain.[2,3,5]
- Colonic tumors: Minor fresh bleeding and occult blood loss is common. The presentation of profuse bleeding may occur.[2,3]
- Angiodysplasia: Vascular anomalies present as multiple lesions in the ascending colon and caecum. Bleeding is commonly slow and intermittent. Hemorrhage can occur with rebleed with endoscopic coagulation of the lesion needed.[2,3]
- Benign anorectal disease: Anorectal lesions, such as hemorrhoids, can present as a hemorrhage.[3]
- Iatrogenic hemorrhage: Hemorrhage may occur after a polypectomy.[3]

ENHANCED FOCUS ON COMMON ACUTE UPPER GASTROINTESTINAL BLEEDING DISORDERS
Peptic Ulcer Disorder

Gastroduodenal ulcers are common causes of upper gastrointestinal bleeding.[3] Defects in the gastric or duodenal mucosa extend deep into the wall, leaving the mucosa vulnerable for breakdown with resultant bleeding.[4,6] Four major risk factors for bleeding are associated with peptic ulcer disease. Elimination of these risk factors reduces ulcer reoccurrence and rebleeding rates.[4,6] These 4 risk factors include

1. *H pylori* infection
   - A spiral bacterium
   - Infects the superficial gastric mucosa
   - Disrupts the mucosal layer
   - Makes the mucosa more susceptible to acid damage
   - Chronic inflammation leads to gastritis
   - Altered gastric secretion and tissue damage leads to peptic ulcer disease[3,4,6]
2. NSAIDs
   - NSAIDs, including low-dose aspirin, predispose ulceration
   - Factor for nonhealing ulcers
   - Recurrent ulcers and complications[3,7,8]
3. Physiologic stress
   - Associated with life events and psychological factors[3,8]
4. Excess gastric acid
   - Impairment of mucosal integrity, leading to cell membrane permeability

- Results in intramural acidosis, cell death, and ulceration
- Control of acid is essential.[3,8]

Major clinical manifestations of peptic ulcer disorder

Major clinical manifestations of peptic ulcer disorder include dyspepsia, silent ulcers, ulcer complications, penetration and fistulation, perforation, and gastroesophageal reflux. Assessment information about these potential manifestations includes

1. Dyspepsia: Eighty percent of patients have epigastric pain with upper abdominal pain most prominent. Duodenal ulcer pain occurs 2 to 5 hours after a meal when acid is secreted. The circadian height of acid secretion is between 11 PM and 2 AM, causing ulcer pain at night.[2,4,8]
2. Asymptomatic: Seventy percent of patients with silent ulcers are asymptomatic. Patients have symptoms when complications and bleeding ulcers occur.[2,4,8]
3. Ulcer complications: Patients with bleeding ulcers present with nausea, red blood or coffee ground emesis, or black tarry stool (hematemesis or melena). Patients with massive bleeding may present with orthostatic hypotension and red or maroon blood in the stool (hematochezia).[4–6] Gastric outlet obstruction can occur if the ulcer is located in the duodenum or pyloric channel.[4] Patients with gastric outlet present with epigastric pain, weight loss, early satiety, bloating, nausea, vomiting, and indigestion.[4,8,9]
4. Penetration and fistulation: Ulcers that penetrate through the bowel wall and adjacent structures present with intense and longer pain duration in the lower thoracic or upper spinal region.[8,9] Penetrating posterior ulcers present with localized back pain that is intense and not relieved with antacids or food.[2,8,9] Gastric or duodenal fistulas present with weight loss, dyspepsia, feculent vomiting, halitosis, and diarrhea.[8,9] Erosion into vascular structures and abscess can lead to hemorrhage.[8,9] Pancreatic duct fistulation can occur with duodenal ulcers.[8,9]
5. Perforation: Duodenal ulcers cause 60% of ulcer perforations. Patients with a perforation present with sudden acute diffuse abdominal pain.[8,9]
6. Associated symptoms: Gastroesophageal reflux is frequently associated with peptic ulcers. Forty-six percent of patients have acid regurgitation and heartburn.[3,8,9]

The cause and bleeding site must be identified to stop the bleeding and empower hemodynamic stability. Common diagnosis and testing include

1. Upper endoscopy: Endoscopy is the standard for diagnosing peptic ulcer disease and 90% accurate in detecting gastroduodenal lesions.[2,8] Benign ulcers are a flat smooth ulcer with smooth, rounded edges.[2,8] Some patients with bleeding ulcers will stop bleeding while hospitalized, whereas some patients will be critical with recurrent hemorrhage.[2,4,8,9]
2. Imaging: Barium radiography is not commonly used because of the radiation to patients and the inability to biopsy a lesion. In imaging, an ulcer is round and surrounded by edema.[4]
3. Test for H pylori: Patients diagnosed with peptic ulcer should be tested for H pylori infection with a biopsy with upper endoscopy.[6] Because of possible false-negative results, testing should be delayed if the patient has acute bleeding, is taking an antibiotic, or is on a proton pump inhibitor. Urea breath test or a stool H pylori antigen test can be used. If the patient is positive, eradiation of the infection should be done.[4,6]

4. Assessment of NSAID use: Assess for history of NSAIDs and low-dose aspirin as a causative factor.[4,7]
5. Differential diagnosis: Diagnostic evaluation should be done to rule out other causes of clinical manifestations of peptic ulcer, such as celiac disease or chronic pancreatitis.[4,7,8]

Treatment of bleeding ulcers

Some patients with bleeding ulcers stop bleeding while hospitalized, whereas some patients are critical with recurrent hemorrhage, in which case interventional angiography or surgery is necessary.[9]

The nurse must use clinical reasoning in developing a plan of care for treatment of unstable patients with bleeding ulcers. Management of bleeding ulcers includes

1. Initial assessment: The initial assessment includes evaluating hemodynamic stability and determining the need for blood transfusion or fluid resuscitation based on clinical presentation and laboratory findings.[4,9] Hemoglobin and hematocrit levels are used to assess gastrointestinal bleeding. During the first 4 to 6 hours, these laboratory values will be in normal range due to time needed for the body to shift fluids to the intravascular compartment.[4,9] The patient should be started on an intravenous proton pump inhibitor during the initial evaluation.[4,9] Acid suppression with treatment by a proton pump inhibitor is recommended for all bleeding ulcer patients. The proton pump inhibitor stabilizes blood clots by elevating gastric pH levels.[4,9] Pantoprazole and esomeprazole are examples of common intravenous formulations that are initially given twice a day with tapering to daily administration. When there is no evidence of bleeding, the patient is switched to an oral proton pump inhibitor such as omeprazole.[4,9] Patients at high risk for bleeding are given a high-dose continuous proton pump inhibitor.[4,9] Coordination of care should be established during initial assessment to develop a collaborative team approach. If the patient is unable, the intensive care team should consult with the gastroenterologist.[4,9,10]
2. Endoscopic therapy: Endoscopy is performed to diagnose a bleeding ulcer. If the ulcer base is not clean, the patient is at risk for recurrent bleeding and the ulcer is classified as high-risk stigmata. The risk classification score provides information about the risk of recurrent bleeding and treatment needed.[3,9] Patients with high risk for recurrent bleeding are hospitalized.[9] Several types of endoscopic therapy are available, depending on the classification of the bleeding ulcer. Most patients are treated with either hemostatic clips or thermal coagulation combined with injection therapy.[4,9–11]
   - Injection therapy: Erythromycin may be given intravenously before the endoscopy in patients with a large amount of blood in their stomach. This medication helps empty out the blood in the stomach, therefore helping with visualization of the stomach during endoscopy.[4,9] Diluted epinephrine injection can stop or reduce bleeding by causing a vasospasm and local tamponade. Injection therapy is used in conjunction with another therapy.[4,9]
   - Thermal coagulation: Contact probes compress the vessel while coagulation is performed to stop bleeding and seal the vessel to prevent recurrent bleeding.[4,9]
   - Hemoclips: Hemoclips are applied during endoscopy for coagulation. Hemoclips are similar to surgical ligation and, if surgery or interventional angiographic is needed, the hemoclips can serve as a radiopaque marker.[9,11,12]
   - Fibrin sealant: During the endoscopic procedure, a fibrin sealant is injected to decrease bleeding.[4,9]

- Hemostatic nanopowder: Nanopowder is sprayed onto the bleeding site through a catheter during the endoscopy procedure. The nanopowder becomes an adhesive when in contact with blood. It also helps clot formation.[4,9,13]
- Second-look endoscopy: The gastroenterologist may want to schedule a follow-up endoscopy within 24 hours of the initial intervention to look for rebleeding.[9,14]
- Endoscopy complications: The nurse needs to assess for complications before and after the emergency endoscopy. A change of condition with clinical manifestations from any of these complications should be reported immediately and rapid response initiated if needed depending on the critical setting. Focused preintervention assessment for clinical manifestations includes aspiration, hypoventilation from over sedation, and hypotension due to inadequate blood transfusion and volume replacement.[10,11,15] Focused postintervention assessment for clinical manifestations of perforation, epinephrine induced tachycardia and arrhythmias, and persistent or recurring bleeding.[10,15] A change in patient condition using clinical reasoning should be reported immediately.
- Surgery: Failed endoscopic therapy and interventional angiography require patients to have surgery for peptic ulcer hemorrhage, hemodynamic instability after 3 blood transfusion units, shock, or perforation. Examples of surgery include oversewing of ulcer, truncal vagotomy, pyloroplasty, and selective vagotomy.[9,10,15]
- Interventional angiography: Rates between 52% and 98% are considered successful for angiography with transarterial embolization for acute peptic ulcer bleeding.[3,9,15]

Resumption of anticoagulants, antiplatelet agents, and nonsteroidal antiinflammatory drugs

All patients need to be evaluated about the risk of bleeding ulcers with resumption of anticoagulants, antiplatelet agents, and NSAIDs. The physician will need to explore the risks with resumption, including a thromboembolic event while off the medication, a new cardiovascular event, and arthritic pain.[16–18] Emergency readmission can occur with rebleeding ulcers caused by continuation of medications associated with bleeding ulcers.[9,16] An informed mutual decision will need to be made between the physician and the patient (or their legal representative).

Case report AJ is a 28-year-old healthy woman. Over the past week she complained of weakness, fatigue, and loss of appetite. On Friday evening she suddenly experienced diarrhea with recurrent episodes of black semiliquid stools. After 3 hours of passing back stools she complained of dizziness, severe weakness, and feeling like she was going to pass out. Her mother took her to the emergency room. Her medication history revealed she had severe menstrual cramps and was prescribed Motrin 800 mg orally 3 times a day. AJ stated she had taken this high prescription dose for 6 months. She was not eating or drinking 8 ounces of fluid with the dose due to loss of appetite. Her hematocrit was 25 and hemoglobin was 9. Radiograph revealed a 5 cm peptic ulcer. She was hospitalized to provide fluid resuscitation and administer an intravenous proton inhibitor. The next morning, AJ was stabilized and discharged from the hospital with a prescription for Prevacid and iron. AJ was instructed to stop the prescription Motrin, avoid spicy food, and return to the emergency room if bleeding reoccurred. An appointment was scheduled the next day with a gastroenterologist for endoscopy and treatment of a peptic ulcer secondary to nonsteroidal medication.

Acute Variceal Hemorrhage

Upper gastrointestinal bleeding from varices is caused by portal hypertension associated with advanced liver disease. Varices may be in the esophagus, stomach, or small bowel.[3,18,19] Gastrointestinal bleeding is due to rupture of collateral portal-systemic encephalopathy or complication of cirrhosis. Rupture leads to with high mortality due to difficulty with controlling the bleeding.[3,18,19]

Common clinical manifestations for varices

Common clinical manifestations for acute variceal hemorrhage include bleeding, hypovolemia, anemia, and cirrhosis, and liver disease. Assessment information about these potential manifestations includes

- Bleeding presents as hematemesis, melena, or hematochezia.
- Hypovolemia and anemia presents as lightheadedness, weakness, tachycardia, and cold hands or feet.
- Cirrhosis presents as ascites, encephalopathy, and jaundice.
- Liver disease presents as spider angiomata.[3,19]

Management of acute variceal hemorrhage

Active bleeding of a ruptured varices is a medical emergency due to hemodynamic instability. Management for active bleeding includes

- Admit to critical care unit
- Protect airway from aspiration and massive bleeding with endotracheal intubation
- Insert nasogastric tube for subsequent endoscopic procedure
- Begin volume resuscitation with crystalloids conservatively if patient has renal failure
- Transfuse red blood cell to maintain hemoglobin with avoidance of mismatched transfusions
- Use fresh frozen plasma to correct coagulopathy
- Start vasoactive medication, such as octreotide or vapreotide
- Start prophylaxis antibiotic, such as norfloxacin or ciprofloxacin
- Administer lactulose for hepatic encephalopathy
- Monitor alcohol withdrawal symptoms and administer thiamine replacement
- Perform an esophagogastroendoscopy within 12 hours to confirm and treat bleeding varices with endoscopic variceal ligation or sclerotherapy
- Perform a transjugular intrahepatic portocaval shunt procedure for continued or recurrent bleeding
- Use a balloon tamponade temporarily for uncontrolled bleeding
- Order a prophylaxis beta blocker, such as nadolol or propranolol, for common recurring bleeding.[20,21]

Case report BW is a 68-year-old man with a history of active alcoholism, cirrhosis, and ascites. He was brought to the emergency room via ambulance after a 911 call. He complained of hematemesis and hematochezia for 4 days, lightheadedness, weakness, and heart racing. His hematocrit was 24, hemoglobin 5.8, blood pressure 86/49, and heart rate 150. BW was resuscitated with fluids and red blood cell packs. When BW was hemodynamically stable, he underwent an urgent upper gastrointestinal endoscopy. The diagnostic test revealed an oozing bleeding varix located at the second portion of the duodenum. Endoscopic variceal band ligation successfully controlled the bleeding. He was diagnosed with an acute variceal bleed. BW returned to his room and was discharged 5 days later after monitoring for recurrent bleeding.

General Management of Acute Upper Gastrointestinal Bleeding

Patients with acute upper gastrointestinal bleeding typically present with hematemesis or melena. The patient may have scant bleeding to profuse bleeding, which requires a critical care setting. The critical care nurse must be knowledgeable about acute upper gastrointestinal bleeding and possess the clinical reasoning skills to intervene on a life-threatening change of condition with hemodynamic instability secondary to a hemorrhagic bleeding episode. General management for these critically ill patients includes

- Triage patient to the appropriate level of care
- Take a medication history with focus on cause of bleeding, such as NSAIDs, aspirin, antiplatelet agents, or anticoagulants
- Take a medical history, including alcohol abuse, liver disease, previous bleed, peptic ulcer disease, renal disease, or heart failure
- Examine for bleeding symptoms, hypovolemia, shock, or abdominal pain; rectal examination for bleeding
- Order laboratory tests, including complete blood count, serum chemistry, liver tests, coagulation studies, electrocardiogram with cardiac enzymes, and serial hemoglobin (this will start at baseline, then go down, and blood urea nitrogen will be elevated with upper bleeding); perform nasogastric lavage to clean stomach before endoscopy
- Triage and consult; with active bleeding, consult with gastroenterology; with perfuse bleeding, consult with interventional radiology
- Resuscitate fluid; observe for fluid overload and bolus
- Transfuse blood, including red blood cells, fresh frozen plasma, and platelets
- Prepare for diagnostic tests; upper endoscopy is standard.[15,16,18,22,23]

ENHANCED FOCUS ON COMMON LOWER GASTROINTESTINAL BLEEDING DISORDERS
Colonic Diverticular Bleeding

Colonic diverticular disorder is the most common cause of lower gastrointestinal bleeding. In the past, this disorder was treated with urgent colectomy but now endoscopy and interventional radiology has transformed the management of colonic diverticular bleeding.[24,25]

Pathogenic changes responsible for bleeding colonic diverticula in the right colon include

- Penetrating vessel ruptures, causing weakness of the wall
- The wall draping over the dome of the diverticulum
- The wall is separated from the bowel lumen by mucosa
- The vasa recta has recurrent injury along its luminal aspect
- Recurrent segmented weakness of the artery
- The artery is at risk to rupture into the lumen.[24,25]

Clinical manifestations
The typical presentation is painless hematochezia. The patient may have self-limited bleeding that stops or massive persistent bleeding. The patient may complain of bloating, cramping, and the urge to defecate due to bleeding serving as a cathartic. Severe bleeding causes hemodynamic instability with the presentation of hypotension or

tachycardia, and may alter level of consciousness.[16,24,25] Initial priority management is resuscitation with fluids, blood products, and correcting coagulopathies.[16,24,25]

Diagnostic testing
The gold standard for identification of the bleeding site in lower gastrointestinal bleeding is the colonoscopy. Diagnostic testing for diverticular bleeding includes

- Nasogastric lavage may be ordered to rule out upper bleeding.
- Colonoscopy is standard for diagnosis. If the bleeding site is identified, banding or endoscopic hemoclips are used to control bleeding.
- If colonoscopy fails, a tagged red cell scan is performed followed by angiography with infusion of a vasoconstriction medication, such as diluted epinephrine.
- If bleeding is not stopped or controlled, a segmented or subtotal colectomy is performed.[23-26]

Angiodysplasias
Angiodysplasias are dilated tortuous submucosal veins found in the gastrointestinal tract that includes the colon, small intestine, stomach, and duodenum. These aberrant vascular blood vessels can cause bleeding at multiple sites.[27-29] They are the most common vascular anomalies found in the gastrointestinal tract, appearing as small flat cherry-red radiating from a central vessel with a fern-like pattern.[27] Conditions associated with angiodysplasias include older age, end stage renal disease, von Willebrand, and aortic stenosis.[27-29] When started, recurrent bleeding is a complication.[27]

Diagnosis and management
Angiodysplasias are usually diagnosed during gastrointestinal bleeding or during a routine colonoscopy. A variety of endoscopic treatments can be used to treat these aberrant vessels, including

- Mechanical measures, such as banding and endoscopic clips
- Argon plasma coagulation
- Electrocoagulation
- Injection of sclerosant
- Argon and neodymium-doped yttrium aluminium garnet (Nd:YAG) lasers.[27-29]

If endoscopic procedures are ineffective, the procedures that may be instituted include

- Computed tomography (CT) angiography
- Angiography with infusion of vasopressin
- Surgery for resection of lesions
- Hormonal therapy with estrogen to control bleeding in small bowel.[27-30]

General Management of Acute Lower Gastrointestinal Bleeding

Patients with acute lower gastrointestinal bleeding typically present with hematochezia and can have self-limiting bleeding or have hemorrhaging that is life-threatening. The critical care nurse must be knowledgeable about acute lower gastrointestinal bleeding and possess the clinical skills to manage these patients in a potential bleeding crisis. General management for these critically ill patients includes

- Triage the patient to the appropriate level of care
- History taking for prior episodes of bleeding, past medical history, medication use, comorbidities, and bleeding symptoms

- Physical examination for signs of hypovolemia and presence of abdominal pain
- Laboratory testing, including complete blood count, serum chemistries, liver tests, and coagulation studies (hemoglobin blood series will be normal then decrease; blood urea nitrogen is normal in lower bleeding)
- Nasogastric lavage to rule out upper bleed (bright red blood or coffee ground blood will be found in lavage fluid if upper bleeding)
- Triage and consultation with gastroenterology for acute bleeding, and general surgery and interventional radiology for massive hematochezia
- Supportive measures, such as supplemental oxygen
- Fluid resuscitation and bolus (intensive monitoring if risk fluid overload)
- Blood transfusions, including red blood and fresh frozen plasma if needed
- Preparation for diagnostic tests; colonoscopy is standard.[16,28,29,31–33]

SUMMARY

A patient with acute gastrointestinal bleeding can have a sudden, radial change in condition from stability to hemodynamic instability with signs of profuse bleeding, shock, and altered mental status. The frontline critical nurse must learn self-efficacy for implementing standards of care for patients with acute gastrointestinal bleeding and have the clinical skills for management of a medical crisis if it occurs. Important skills to remember are (1) triaging the patient to the appropriate level of care with protection of the patient's airway because of the profuse hematemesis with mechanical ventilation, (2) fluid resuscitation with monitoring signs of fluid overload, (3) critical review of serial hemoglobin levels and ordering other blood tests, (4) blood transfusions, (5) preparing patient for urgent or emergency diagnostic tests, and (6) developing a collaborative team approach for consults with a gastroenterologist, interventional radiologist, and surgeon. This article overviewed upper and lower acute gastrointestinal bleeding and provided current evidence-based standards of care for nursing management of acute gastrointestinal bleeding. Common bleeding disorders were reviewed with expanded focus on peptic ulcer, acute variceal hemorrhage, colonic diverticular bleeding, and angiodysplasias, which are commonly found in the critical care setting. The standards of care for these common bleeding disorders provide a skills toolkit for managing patients with acute gastrointestinal bleeding disorders and managing a medical emergency that can save patients' lives.

REFERENCES

1. Thompson DG. Structure and function of the gut. In: Warrell DA, Cox TM, Firth JS, editors. Oxford textbook of medicine. 5th edition. Oxford (United Kingdom): Oxford University Press; 2010. p. 2201–4.

2. Leary S. Gastrointestinal disorders and therapeutic management. In: Urden RD, Stacy KM, Lough ME, editors. Critical care nursing diagnosis and management. 7th edition. St Louis (MO): Elsevier; 2014. p. 751–63.

3. Rockall TA, Dawson HM. Gastrointestinal bleeding. In: Warrell DA, Cox TM, Firth JS, editors. Oxford textbook of medicine. 5th edition. Oxford (United Kingdom): Oxford University Press; 2010. p. 2233–7.

4. Sung J. Peptic ulcer disease. In: Warrell DA, Cox TM, Firth JS, editors. Oxford textbook of medicine. 5th edition. Oxford (United Kingdom): Oxford University Press; 2010. p. 2305–15.

5. Center for Disease Control and Prevention. Helicobacter pylori. 1998. Available at: www.cdc.gov/ncidod/dbmd/hpylori.htm. Accessed June 5, 2017.

6. Jewell DP. Ulcerative colitis. In: Warrell DA, Cox TM, Firth JS, editors. Oxford textbook of medicine. 5th edition. Oxford (United Kingdom): Oxford University Press; 2010. p. 2371–83.

7. Hreinsson JP, Palsdottir S, Bjornsson ES. The association of drugs with severity and specific causes of acute gastrointestinal bleeding a prospective study. J Clin Gastroenterol 2016;50(5):408–13. Available at: www.jcge.com. Accessed June 5, 2017.

8. Vakil NB, Feldman M, Grover S, editors. Peptic ulcer disease: clinical manifestations and diagnosis. 2017. Available at: www.uptodate.com. Accessed June 15, 2017.

9. Saltzman JR, Feldman M, Travis AC, editors. Overview of the treatment of bleeding peptic ulcers. 2017. Available at: www.uptodate.com. Accessed June 15, 2017.

10. Vakil NB, Feldman M, Grover S, editors. Overview of the complications of peptic ulcer disease. 2017. Available at: www.uptodate.com. Accessed June 15, 2017.

11. Wang J, Hu D, Tang W, et al. Simple risk factors to predict urgent endoscopy in nonvariceal upper gastrointestinal Bleeding pre-endoscopically. Medicine 2016; 95(26):1–6.

12. Wander P, Castaneda D, Carr-Locke D. Single center experience of an endoscopic clip in managing nonvariceal upper gastrointestinal bleeding. J Clin Gastroenterol 2017;0(0):1–6. Available at: www.jcge.com. Retrieved June 10, 2017.

13. Preib J, Barmeyer C, Burgel N, et al. Hemostatic system in nonvariceal gastrointestinal bleeding results of a prospective multicenter observational pilot study. J Clin Gastroenterol 2016;30(10):95–100. Available at: www.jcge. Accessed June 10, 2017.

14. Imperiale TF, Kong N. Second-look endoscopy for bleeding peptic ulcer disease A decision-effectiveness and cost-effectiveness analysis. J Clin Gastroenterol 2012;46(9):71–5. Available at: www.jcge.com. Accessed June 10, 2017.

15. Cooper K. Disorders of the stomach. In: Cooper K, Gasnell K, editors. Adult health nursing. 7th edition. St Louis (MO): Elsevier; 2015. p. 192–202.

16. Day M. Gastrointestinal bleeding. In: Carlson K, editor. AACN advanced critical care nursing. 1st edition. St Louis (MO): Saunders Elsevier; 2009. p. 737–46.

17. Sostres C, Lanas A. Should prophylactic low-dose aspirin therapy be continued in peptic ulcer bleeding? Drugs 2011;71(1):1–9.

18. DeWit S, Stromberg H, Dallred C. The gastrointestinal system. In: Medical-surgical nursing. 3rd edition. St Louis (MO): Elsevier; 2017. p. 624–43.

19. Stromdahl M, Helgeson J, Kalaitzakis E. Emergency readmission following acute upper gastrointestinal bleeding. Eur J Gastroenterol Hepatol 2017;29:73–7.

20. Jackson CS, Fedorowicz Z, Oettgen P, editors. Acute variceal hemorrhage. 2013. Available at: http://dynmed.com. Accessed June 10, 2017.

21. Sanyal AJ, Runyon BA, Robson KM, editors. General principles of the management of variceal hemorrhage. Available at: www.uptodate.com. Accessed June 10, 2017.

22. Saltzman JA, Feldman M, Travis AC, editors. Approach to acute upper gastrointestinal bleeding in adults. 2017. Available at: www.uptodate.com. Accessed June 10, 2017.

23. Krumberger JM. How to manage an acute upper GI bleed. RN 2005;26(3):34–9.

24. Pemberton JH, Saltzman JR, Grover S, editors. Colonic diverticular bleeding. 2017. Available at: www.uptodate.com. Accessed June 10, 2017.

25. Cirocchi R, Grassi V, Cavaliere D, et al. New trends in acute management of colonic diverticular bleeding: a systematic review. Medicine 2015;94(44):1–7.

26. Williams CB, Saunders BP. Colonoscopy and flexible sigmoidoscopy. In: Warrell DA, Cox TM, Firth JS, editors. Oxford textbook of medicine, 5th edition. Oxford (United Kingdom): Oxford University Press; 2010. p. 2210–3.
27. Pedrosa MC, Friedman LS, Travis AC, editors. Angiodysplasia of the Gastrointestinal Tract. Available at: www.uptodate.com. Accessed June 10, 2017.
28. Strate LL, Grainek IM. Management of patients with acute lower gastrointestinal bleeding. Am J Gastroenterol 2016;111(4):459–74.
29. Gralnek LM, Neeman Z, Strate LL. Acute lower gastrointestinal bleeding. N Engl J Med 2017;376(11):1054–63.
30. Garcia-Blazquez V, Vicente-Bartulos A, Olavarria-Delgado A, et al. Emergency Radiology Accuracy of CT angiography in the diagnosis of acute gastrointestinal bleeding: systematic review and meta-analysis. Eur Radiol 2013;23:1181–90.
31. Currie GM, Kiat H, Wheat JM. Scintigraphic evaluation of acute lower gastrointestinal hemorrhage current status and future directions. J Clin Gastroenterol 2011; 45(2):92–9.
32. Hashash JG, Shamseddeen W, Skoury A, et al. Gross lower gastrointestinal bleeding in patients on anticoagulants and/or antiplatelet therapy endoscopic findings, managements, and clinical outcomes. J Clin Gastroenterol 2007; 43(1):36–42.
33. Edelman DA, Sugawa C. Lower gastrointestinal bleeding: a review. Surg Endosc 2007;21(4):514–20.

Acute Diverticulitis Management

Deborah L. Ellison, PhD, MSN, BSN

KEYWORDS

- Diverticular disease • Acute diverticulitis • Pathogenesis • Medical management
- Surgical management

KEY POINTS

- Acute diverticulitis is a painful disease that represents inflammation and can require hospitalization and/or surgery.
- Diverticular disease is characterized by the presence of saclike protrusions (diverticula) in the colonic mucosa.
- Diverticulitis is defined as an inflammation of the diverticulum, and can be asymptomatic or symptomatic.
- Abdominal pain is the most common complaint in patients with acute diverticulitis.

INTRODUCTION

Acute diverticulitis is a painful disease that represents inflammation and can require hospital and/or surgery (**Tables 1–3**). The diverticulum is a saclike protrusion of the colonic or bowel wall.[1] Diverticulosis is defined by the presence of diverticula. Diverticular disease is characterized by the presence of diverticula in the colonic mucosa. Diverticular disease accounts for approximately 300,000 hospitalizations per year in the United States, resulting in 1.5 million days of inpatient care.[2] Diverticulitis is defined as an inflammation of the diverticulum, which can be asymptomatic or symptomatic. Acute diverticulitis is defined as inflammation, generally considered to be caused by microperforation of a diverticulum.[3] Diverticulitis can further be categorized as chronic or acute, uncomplicated or complicated, depending on the extent of the complications of the diverticular. The exact cause is unknown but it is associated with age greater than 60 years, decreased dietary fiber, increased intracolonic pressure, abnormal neuromuscular function, and alterations in intestinal mobility.[4]

This disease is the third most common gastrointestinal illness that requires hospitalization and the leading indication for elective colon resection.[5,6,7] In Western and industrialized societies, diverticular disease is a significant contributor to health care

Disclosure: The author has no commercial or financial conflicts of interest or any funding sources.
Austin Peay State University, School of Nursing, 601 College Street, Clarksville, TN 37043, USA
E-mail address: ellisond@apsu.edu

Table 1
Plan of care for conservative outpatient management

Problems	Interventions
Infection and pain	Diagnostics (completed in the emergency room) • CT scan with oral and intravenous contrast • CBC with differential and serum electrolytes Collaborative therapy • Bed rest • Analgesics (acetaminophen, ibuprofen, or oxycodone) • Clear liquid diet • Reschedule a clinic visit in 2 to 3 d

Abbreviations: CBC, complete blood count; CT, computed tomography.
Data from Refs.[1,11,12]

costs because of the increase in prevalence of diverticulosis; 5% to 25% of patients develop diverticulitis and 5% to 15% develop symptomatic bleeding.[7,8,9] The mean age of admission for acute diverticulitis is 63 years.[3] Nevertheless, with the increase in incidence, patients with acute diverticulitis can present at 45 years of age or even earlier.[10]

Many of these patients are admitted to a critical care unit because of the risk of bleeding and other complications. Critical care nurses are on the frontline of health care and must have the knowledge, skills, and attitudes to care for patients with acute diverticulitis. This article provides critical care nurses with the specialized knowledge

Table 2
Critical care nursing plan of care for inpatient management

Problem and Complications	Interventions

Infection, pain, possible peritonitis, hypovolemic shock, sepsis	Diagnostics
	• CT scan with oral and intravenous contrast (repeat on admission)
	• CBC with differential and serum electrolytes (repeat on admission)
	Collaborative therapy
	• Nursing assessment (vital signs every hour, abdominal assessment to include quality and presence of bowel sounds, abdominal distention, abdominal guarding, nausea, fever)
	• IV antibiotic therapy
	• NPO status initially, slowly moving to clear liquids with improvement
	• NG suctioning
	• IV fluids (normal saline or Ringer lactate)
	• Strict I/O
	• Bed rest
	• Analgesics (morphine, ketorolac, or hydromorphone)
	• Surgery
	  ○ Possible resection of involved colon for obstruction or hemorrhage
	  ○ Possible temporary colostomy

Abbreviations: I/O, intake/output; IV, intravenous; NG, nasogastric; NPO, nil by mouth.
Data from Refs.[1,11,12]

Table 3 Discharge teaching and patient education	
Discharge Instructions	**Patient Education**
Diet	• Increase fiber; fruits and vegetables are a good source. High fiber includes prunes, baked beans, kidney and lima beans, lentils, oats, peas, and green leafy vegetables • Decrease intake of fat and red meat • Do not have to avoid nuts, seeds, or corn • Inability to tolerate fluids
Complications	• Watch for bloody or dark maroon stools • Increase in abdominal pain, distention, or tenderness • Avoid intra-abdominal pressure (may precipitate attacks), straining with stool, vomiting, bending, lifting, and wearing tight restrictive clothing • Monitor for fever >37.8°C (100.1°F) • Complete all medications as instructed
Activity	• Increase activity as tolerated • Weight reduction

Data from Schmelzer M. Lower gastrointestinal problems. In: Lewis SL, Dirksen SR, Heitkemper MM, et al. editors. Medical surgical nursing: assessment and management of clinical problems. 9th edition. St Louis: Elsevier Mosby; 2014. p. 961-1003; and Pemberton JH. Patient education: diverticular disease (Beyond the Basics). Available at: https://www.uptodate.com/contents/diverticular-disease-beyond-the-basics. Accessed June 1 2017.

of treatment plans, surgical procedures, pain management, and complications to care for patients with acute diverticulitis. This article also includes a nursing focus on older adults with diverticulitis.

Pathophysiology

Diverticulitis predominantly involves the left colon, whereas the right colon is the source of diverticular bleeding in 50% to 90% of patients.[4,8] It rarely occurs in the small intestines.[4] The diverticula form at the weak points in the colon wall, which is usually where arteries penetrate the tunica muscular to nourish the mucosal layer.[4,7] The colonic mucosa herniates through the smooth muscle layers, as shown in **Fig. 1**. Additional structural changes, such as thickening of the circular and longitudinal (teniae coli) muscles surrounding the diverticula, is common in sigmoid diverticula.[4,7] Hypertrophy and contraction of the muscles increase intraluminal pressure and the degree of herniation and could be explained by consumption of a low-residue diet, which reduces fecal bulk, thus reducing the diameter of the colon.[17] In addition, the Laplace law can explain the diverticula in the sigmoid colon. According to the Laplace law, wall pressure increases as the diameter of a cylindrical structure decreases.[4,7] Because the sigmoid colon is the segment of colon with the smallest diameter, pressure within the area can increase enough to rupture the diverticula.

Clinical Manifestations

Although symptoms of diverticular disease are usually vague or absent for years, the clinical presentation of acute diverticulitis depends on the severity of the underlying inflammatory process and the presence of associated complications.[3] Abdominal pain is the most common complaint in patients with acute diverticulitis. The pain can be described as cramping, constant, and persistent for several days. The only exception is in the Asian population, in which the pain may occur on the right

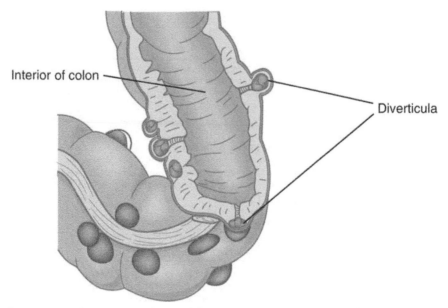

Interior of colon

Diverticula

Fig. 1. Diverticula are outpouchings of the colon. When they become inflamed, the condition is diverticulitis. The inflammatory process can spread to the surrounding area in the intestine. (*From* Schmelzer M. Lower gastrointestinal problems. In: Lewis SL, Dirksen SR, Heitkemper MM, et al, editors. Medical surgical nursing: assessment and management of clinical problems. 9th edition. St Louis: Elsevier Mosby; 2014. p. 995; with permission.)

side.[4,7] Additional symptoms include nausea and vomiting, fever, abdominal tenderness, and constipation (or, less commonly, diarrhea).[3,4]

Medical Management

In acute diverticulitis the overarching goal of treatment is to let the colon rest and the inflammation diminish.[11] Acute diverticulitis can be medically managed either by inpatient or outpatient care, or inpatient care with surgical intervention. Criteria for inpatients include:

- Computed tomography (CT) shows complicated diverticulitis with perforation, abscess, obstruction, or fistulization.
- CT shows uncomplicated diverticulitis but the patient presents with 1 or more of the following:
  - Sepsis
  - High fever (>39.2°C [102.5°F])
  - Immunosuppression (eg, poorly controlled diabetes, advanced human immunodeficiency virus)
  - Significant leukocytosis
  - Severe abdominal pain or diffuse peritonitis
  - Advanced age
  - Significant comorbidities
  - Intolerance of oral intake
  - Noncompliance/unreliability for return visits/lack of support system
  - Failed outpatient treatment.[11,12]

Case Presentation

The following case study presents the medical management of a patient with acute diverticulitis as the patient goes from outpatient to inpatient care through an algorithm.

K. E. is a 47-year-old white woman who presents to the emergency room with complaints of severe left lower abdominal pain. She states that, "It started a week or so ago but has progressively gotten worse; something is wrong." K. E. takes no medication and has no past medical history. Vital signs are stable at this time. CT of the abdomen indicates acute colonic diverticulitis with microperforation that is walled off at this time.

Does the patient meet any of the criteria for inpatient management?[12] No, not at this time. The patient will be managed as an outpatient and prescribed the oral antibiotics ciprofloxacin plus metronidazole (most common) for 7 to 10 days and is restricted to a clear liquid diet.[11,12] She is given oxycodone for pain that is unrelieved by ibuprofen.

Additional collaborative management could include a high-fiber diet, dietary fiber supplements, stool softeners, anticholinergics, and weight reduction (if overweight) as this initial episode subsides.[1,11,12]

On day 3, the patient returns to the clinic. Is there clinical improvement? If yes, advance diet to semisoft and reassess in a week, to ensure clinical improvement. If no, admit patient to hospital.[12]

K. E states: "I cannot tolerate liquids; I am so nauseated." K. E. is admitted to the critical care unit. The following plan of care is initiated by the critical care nurse to provide safe, quality, patient-centered care.

It is critical to remember that, if patients (both inpatients and outpatients) do not respond to treatment within 3 to 5 days,[1,11,12] the goal is to have decreased abdominal pain and tenderness, resolution of significant leukocytosis, and the ability to tolerate an oral diet.

Nursing Focus on Older Adults

As previously noted, the average age of patients with acute diverticulitis is 65 years. Americans are living longer, so the incidence of acute diverticulitis will continue to increase. The following list will assist frontline nurses with history, assessments, reevaluation, and education for the elderly population.

- Provide antibiotics, analgesics, and anticholinergics as prescribed. Observe older patients carefully for side effects of these drugs, especially confusion (or increased confusion), urinary retention or failure, and orthostatic hypotension.
- Do not give laxatives or enemas. Teach patients and their families about the importance of avoiding these measures.
- Encourage patients to rest and to avoid activities that may increase intra-abdominal pressure, such as straining and bending.
- While diverticulitis is active, provide a low-fiber diet. When the inflammation resolves, provide a high-fiber diet. Teach the patients and their families about these diets and when they are appropriate.
- Because older patients do not always experience the typical pain or fever expected, observe carefully for other signs of active disease, such as a sudden change in mental status.
- Perform frequent abdominal assessments to determine distention and tenderness on palpation.
- Check stools for occult or frank bleeding.[13,14]

On admission to the hospital, the CT scan is repeated. Is there a frank perforation, obstruction, or fistula? If yes, refer to surgery. If not, is there a drainable abscess? If yes, the abscess needs to be drained. If no, wait for 2 to 3 days to see whether there is any clinical improvement.[12]

K. E. has no perforation, obstruction, fistula, or abscess at this time. It is recommended that medical management be given time to work.

If there is no clinical improvement, repeat the CT scan. Is there a new complication? If no, continue intravenous antibiotics for another 1 or 2 days. If yes, and there is clinical improvement, advance diet and convert to oral antibiotics when tolerating food.[12]

K. E. is showing signs of clinical improvement. She states that the pain and tenderness are better, and she feels a little hungry. Her diet is advanced to clear liquids and, if she tolerates the clear liquids, the nasogastric (NG) tube will be discontinued. The next morning K. E. is doing better. She has had minimal nausea, no vomiting, and the NG tube is removed. After lunch, her diet is advanced to semisoft. By the next morning, K. E. is started on oral antibiotics and transferred to a medical/surgical unit until she has met all discharge criteria. All of the following discharge criteria must be met:

- Normalization of vital signs
- Resolution of severe abdominal pain
- Resolution of significant leukocytosis
- Tolerance of oral diet.[12]

Surgical Management

Although advances in medical management have been made, the need for surgical intervention is still prevalent for patients with recurrent episodes of acute diverticulitis.[9] The treatment of acute diverticulitis depends on the severity of the symptoms and about 10% to 15% of patients require surgery.[12] Acute diverticulitis with frank (free) perforation is life threatening and an indication for emergency surgery.[12] Surgery may be indicated in patients who do not show clinical improvement after 3 to 5 days of intravenous antibiotic therapy or changes on the CT scan, such as abscess that has not responded to treatment, obstruction, or a fistula.

Additional patients who may require or be offered a surgical option include those diagnosed with chronic smoldering diverticulitis, asymptomatic but high-risk patients, patients who had a complicated diverticulitis attack, and those who are immunocompromised.[12] Patients who initially respond to medical treatment but subsequently develop recurrent symptoms in the weeks following treatment may have chronic smoldering diverticulitis. Elective surgery is offered to patients in the last 3 categories as well. These patients with complicated acute diverticulitis can have a life-threatening situation if they have additional episodes.[12]

Surgery techniques for diverticulitis depend on the patient's hemodynamic stability, extent of the peritoneal contamination, and the surgeon's experience.[12] Techniques include resection of the section of colon that is affected and/or reconstructive surgery to restore intestinal continuity if possible. If the patient is too unstable, a laparotomy with limited resection may be chosen. The most commonly performed procedure is a 2-stage procedure called the Hartmann procedure.[12] In the Hartmann procedure the diseased colon section is resected, creating an end colostomy and a rectal stump, followed by reversal of the colostomy 3 months later.[12] There is significant difficulty and high mortality associated with the reversal of the colostomy.[12]

SUMMARY

Diverticulitis is defined as an inflammation of the diverticulum, and can be asymptomatic or symptomatic. This disease is the third most common gastrointestinal illness that requires hospitalization and the leading indication for elective colon resection.

Diverticular disease accounts for approximately 300,000 hospitalizations per year in the United States, resulting in 1.5 million days of inpatient care. Although symptoms of diverticular disease are usually vague or absent for years, abdominal pain is the most common complaint in patients with acute diverticulitis. Critical care nurses must be able to take an accurate health history and a pain assessment.[15,16] The pain can be described as cramping, constant, and persistent for several days. Medical management is most often provided with antibiotics and clear liquid diet. Surgery is complicated and the surgery techniques for diverticulitis depend on the patient's hemodynamic stability, extent of the peritoneal contamination, and the surgeon's experience.[12] Acute diverticulitis is still under-researched in many areas of nutrition and treatment.[17,18]

REFERENCES

1. Milovic V. Small bowel diverticula: clinical manifestations, diagnosis, and management. UpToDate; 2017. Available at: http://www.uptodate.com. Accessed June 1, 2017.
2. Escalante R, Bustamante-Lopez L, Lizcano A, et al. Peritoneal lavage in complicated acute diverticulitis: back to the future. J Clin Gastroenterol 2016;50(1): S83-5.
3. Pemberton JH. Clinical manifestations and diagnosis of acute diverticulitis in adults. UpToDate; 2016. Available at: http://www.uptodate.com. Accessed June 1, 2017.
4. McCance K, Sue H. Pathophysiology: the biologic basis for disease in adults and children, 7th edition. St. Lewis (MO): Mosby; 2015.
5. Peery AF, Dellon ES, Lund J, et al. Burden of gastrointestinal disease in the United States: 2012 update. Gastroenterology 2012;143(5):1179-87.e1-3.
6. Anaya DA, Flum DR. Risk of emergency colectomy and colostomy in patients with diverticular disease. Arch Surg 2005;140(7):681-5.
7. Pemberton JH. Colonic diverticulosis and diverticular disease: epidemiology, risk factors, and pathogenesis. UpToDate; 2017. Available at: http://www.uptodate. com. Accessed June 1, 2017.
8. Dirweesh A, Amodu A, Khan M, et al. Symptomatic diverticular disease in patients with severely reduced kidney function: higher rates of complications and transfusion requirement. Gastroenterology Res 2017;10(1):15-20.
9. Gralista P, Moris D, Vailas M, et al. Laparoscopic approach in colonic diverticulitis: dispelling myths and misperceptions. Surg Laparosc Endosc Percutan Tech 2017;27(2):73-82.
10. Bastiani RD, Sanna G, Francasso P, et al. The management of patients with diverticulosis and diverticular disease in primary care. J Clin Gastroenterol 2016;50(1): S89-92.
11. Schmelzer M. Lower gastrointestinal problems. In: Lewis SL, Dirksen SR, Heitkemper MM, editors. Medical surgical nursing: assessment and management of clinical problems. 9th edition. St Louis: Elsevier Mosby; 2014. p. 961-1003.
12. Pemberton JH. Acute colonic diverticulitis: medical management. UpToDate; 2017. Available at: http://www.uptodate.com. Accessed June 1, 2017.
13. Ignatavicius D, Workman M. Medical-surgical nursing: patient-centered collaborative care. 8th edition. St. Lewis (MO): Saunders; 2016.
14. Pemberton JH. Patient education: diverticular disease (Beyond the Basics). UpToDate; 2016. Available at: http://www.uptodate.com. Accessed June 1, 2017.

15. Urden L, Stacy K, Lough M. Critical care nursing. 7th edition. St. Lewis (MO): Mosby; 2017.
16. Böhm SK. Risk factors for diverticulosis, diverticulitis, diverticular perforation, and bleeding: a plea for more subtle history taking. Viszeralmedizin 2015;31(2): 84–94.
17. Tursi A. Diverticulosis today. Unfashionable and still under-researched. Therap Adv Gastroenterol 2016;9(2):213–28.
18. Elisei W, Tursi A. Recent advances in the treatment of colonic diverticular disease and prevention of acute diverticulitis. Ann Gastroenterol 2016;29(1):24–32.

Educating Nurses in the Intensive Care Unit About Gastrointestinal Complications

Using an Algorithm Embedded into Simulation

Loretta Bond, RN, PhD, CNE, Beth Hallmark, RN, PhD, CHSE*

KEYWORDS

- Algorithm • Rubric • Clinical judgment • Failure to rescue • GI failure
- Intensive care unit • Sequential organ failure assessment (SOFA) • Simulation

KEY POINTS

- Intensive care unit (ICU) nurses can be trained to use their surveillance and clinical judgment skills using an algorithm embedded into simulation education.
- The goal of ICU nurse simulation education is to facilitate the rapid identification of deterioration and subsequent escalation of care in the prevention of failure to rescue (FTR).
- Risk scoring tools, such as the sequential organ failure assessment (SOFA) and gastrointestinal failure (GIF) score are helpful in determining patients at risk for FTR.
- Early recognition of patient deterioration can be assessed in simulation through interpretation of observations collected through the SOFA and GIF scores, and management of care priorities can be applied during the simulation and reflected on during debriefing.
- To prepare ICU nurses to care for complex patients with complex gastrointestinal disorders, the Tanner clinical judgment framework was embedded into an algorithm and applied to educational simulation.

INTRODUCTION

Although the complexity of care in all acute care settings is increasing, the multifaceted needs of patients in the intensive care unit (ICU) are often overwhelming even for experienced nurses[1]. Nurses in the ICU are inundated with high-risk patients who require vigilant observation and complicated care regimes.[2] Nurses must be able to process and analyze both objective and subjective data for timely and aggressive interventions to be implemented. In order to reverse processes that indicate

Disclosure: Both authors attest that there are no financial or commercial conflicts of interest or any funding sources related to this article.
Belmont University-Gordon E. Inman College of Health Sciences & Nursing, 1900 Belmont Boulevard, Nashville, TN 37212-3757, USA
* Corresponding author.
E-mail address: Beth.hallmark@belmont.edu

deterioration and to ensure patient safety, nurses must be adequately prepared to care for at-risk patients. This requirement means that ICU nurses must be trained to use their surveillance and clinical judgment skills. Patients with gastrointestinal (GI) complications are no exception, presenting in the ICU with often vague but serious issues.

In 2016, Makary and Daniel[3] calculated that medical error was the third leading cause of death in the United States (**Fig. 1**). When reporting the causes of deaths in the United States, the Centers for Disease Control and Prevention (CDC) noted that "human and systems factors are not taken into account."[3] Human factors refer to human strengths and limitations in the interactions of systems and environments that may affect performance.[4] Based on these statistics, prevention of deaths related to human factors must be implemented in all areas of the acute care setting.

Background

Among the causes of deaths related to human error is failure to rescue (FTR). FTR occurs when a hospitalized patient dies or incurs a disability from a treatable condition.[1] The complications and deterioration are likely to involve subtle (and sometimes obvious) signs and symptoms that are dismissed as not being concerning or that are missed.[5] The problem is magnified if nurses are not being prepared to recognize the signs and symptoms of the deterioration and there are communication failures between health care providers.[1] In the United States, FTR has become a national problem and is currently being reported as a quality marker.

The Institute for HealthCare Improvement reported the association between early recognition of patient deterioration and a decrease in hospital-related deaths.[6]

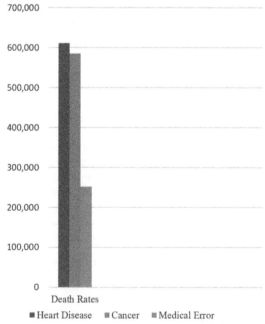

Fig. 1. Death rate 2013. (*Data from* Makary MA, Daniel M. Medical error—the third leading cause of death in the US. BMJ 2016;2139:i2139. doi:10.1136/bmj.i2139.)

Statistics have shown that patients show signs and symptoms of complications and impending arrest as early as 72 hours before an arrest. Reasons for delayed response to patient deterioration are multifaceted and include insufficient resources, inadequate training, poor safety procedures, and poor interpersonal communication.[7] It is critical that, as early signs become evident, nurses are able to identify, report, and intervene to prevent the escalation of deterioration.[8] Among patients who experience unrecognized deterioration in clinical condition leading to unplanned transfer to an ICU, mortalities have been reported to be as high as 50% to 60%.[9]

It is imperative that all health care staff be proficient in the recognition of and response to patient deterioration, and staff should receive training to be able to perform these important skills.[10] This article explores the use of an algorithm embedded into simulation education to develop clinical judgment. Both the sequential organ failure assessment (SOFA; **Table 1**) and GI failure (GIF) tools are integrated for scaffolding assessment skills in the ICU. The role of nurse educators is to prepare the staff to facilitate the rapid identification of deterioration and subsequent escalation of care in the prevention of FTR.

Theoretic Framework

Tanner[11] asserts that the implementation of clinical judgment requires a combination of the knowledge that the nurse brings to the situation, knowledge of the patient and typical patient responses, along with the clinical context and the culture of the nursing unit. Four active processes are applied to sound clinical judgment: noticing, interpreting, responding, and reflection.[11] These 4 processes are the core of clinical judgment and are crucial in complex care situations in which there are continuous changes in patient status and uncertainty about nursing actions.[12] Tanner's[11] clinical judgment model (**Fig. 2**) forms the framework for the development of the clinical judgment and decision making for this article. Patients with GI complications come to the ICU with multidimensional presentations requiring nurses to use the processes of clinical judgment. In order to prepare the ICU nurses to care for patients with complex GI conditions, Tanner's[11] framework and an associated algorithm was developed and applied to educational simulation.

Patients with Gastrointestinal Conditions in the Critical Care Setting

Patients who have GI complications may present in the emergency department or develop complications on a general care unit. Transfer to the ICU is crucial to the care of critically ill patients with GI conditions and is often a vital step in the patient rescue. Because care escalation has already begun on admission to the ICU, early identification of deterioration may be complicated by other symptoms.

Preparing ICU nurses to recognize patients who may have worsening conditions in the midst of the many factors that require the nurses' attention can be a challenge. Patients with GI complications can become gravely ill very rapidly. Identification of deterioration in patients with GI conditions may also be delayed if there are preexisting conditions, such as obesity, advanced age, chronic alcohol use, or altered states such as fluid imbalances and increased hematocrit, blood urea nitrogen level, or creatinine level.[13] In addition, early identification may be complicated by the nature of the pain, which could be referred pain based on the origin of the problem. Other symptoms, such as abdominal distention, hiccups, fever, and pain (especially with rebound tenderness), may be early signs of serious complications. FTR rates increase as the number of complications increases.[14] Because the literature supports the correlation of intestinal failure with organ failure and identifies this relationship as a key determinant of outcomes in critically ill patients, ensuring that nurses are well versed in the

Table 1
Sequential organ failure assessment score

System	0	1	2	3	4
Respiratory P_aO_2/Fio_2 (mm Hg)	≥400 (53.3)	<400 (53.3)	<300 (40)	<200 (26.7)[a]	<100 (13.3)
Platelets (×10³/mL)	≥150	<150	<100	<50	<20
Bilirubin (mg/dL)	1.2	1.2–1.9	2.0–5.9	6.0–11.9	12.0
MAP or Administration of Vasopressors	≥70 mm Hg	<70 mm Hg	Dopamine <5 µg/kg/min or dobutamine	Dopamine 5.1–15 µg/kg/min or adrenaline/noradrenaline ≤0.1 µg/kg/min	Dopamine >15 µg/kg/min or adrenaline/noradrenaline >0.1 µg/kg/min
Glasgow Coma Score	15	13–14	10–12	6–9	<6
Creatinine (mg/dL)	1.2	1.2–1.9	2.0–3.4	3.5–4.9	5.0
UOP (mL/d)	—	—	—	<500	<200

Abbreviations: Fio_2, fraction of inspired oxygen; MAP, mean arterial pressure; UOP, urinary output.

[a] Requires respiratory support.

Data from Vincent JL, Moreno R, Takala J, et al. The SOFA (Sepsis-related Organ Failure Assessment) score to describe organ dysfunction/failure. Intensive Care Med 1996;22(7):707–10.

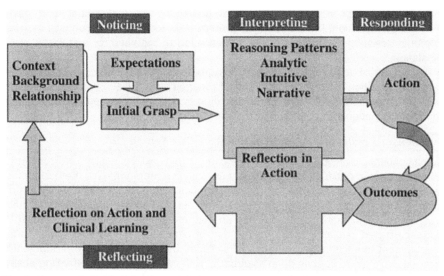

Fig. 2. Tanner clinical judgment model. (*From* Tanner CA. Thinking like a nurse: a research-based model of clinical judgment in nursing. J Nurs Educ 2006;45(6):208; with permission.)

care of patients with GI conditions is imperative to prevent further complications. GIF, when combined with organ failure, is a predictor and risk factor for increased mortality.[15,16]

Risk scoring tools, such as the SOFA[17] and GIF scores, are helpful in determining patients at risk for FTR. The SOFA score is a validated screening tool that measures organ dysfunction (neurologic, blood, liver, kidney, and blood pressure/hemodynamics) and is commonly used to identify risk and predict patient outcomes in acute care settings. The higher the SOFA score, the higher the likelihood of mortality.[17] The SOFA tool (see **Table 1**) is preferred for its simplicity and ease of score calculation.[18] Note that some degree of organ dysfunction necessitating treatment is present in most critically ill patients.[19] The SOFA score tool can be key in the early detection of complications and in the facilitation of care escalation. Attending to standards by nurses and compelling themselves to stick to them are crucial in giving care and could lead to error prevention on their side.[2] Educating nurses to use standard tools is a crucial step in preventing medical error. Scoring systems that can predict GIF may enhance data obtained from the SOFA.[15] Additional assessment criteria, such as intra-abdominal pressure and feeding tolerance, are available to assist nurses as they determine risk for complications.[15,20]

Intra-abdominal hypertension (IAH) is prevalent in about 50% of the critically ill population.[21] The association of IAH and abdominal compression syndrome (ACS) is well documented in acutely ill patients. In addition, both IAH and ACS are associated with multiple organ dysfunction because persistent increased abdominal pressure leads to diminished gut perfusion. Altered perfusion and pressure in the abdominal cavity can lead to necrosis, which can cause bacteria to shift from the GI tract into the blood stream,[13,21,22] especially in individuals who have undergone GI surgery or who have received large-volume fluid resuscitation.[23] When the pressure in the abdominal cavity is sustained at 12 mm Hg or greater the pressure can impede blood flow not only in the gut but in all major body systems, which can lead to multisystem organ failure. Care should be focused on supportive treatment, preventing further distention, and maintaining organ function. Protocols and algorithms that trigger care responses may be helpful in assisting ICU nurses in the identification of the need for aggressive care escalation.

The degree of underlying illness and comorbidities contributes to how rapidly the patient's condition changes. The speed of recognition of these changes by nurses may be determined by the degree of deviation from baseline assessments and the ability of the patients to provide subjective data.[1]

Overview of Simulation Education in the Acute Care Setting

Human patient simulation allows for training of complex skills in realistic environments without exposing patients to unnecessary risk and is a recommended method for the ongoing education and assessment of competence of intensive care nurses.[24] Simulation is an ideal tool for nurturing clinical judgment, to enable practitioners to fully grasp a clinical situation and determine appropriate action based on the context.[12] Evidence-based research supports the use of simulation for nursing professional development to enhance knowledge and skills, as well as confidence development.[6] Professional confidence has been associated with increased decision-making ability and decreased 30-day mortalities. In addition, enhanced confidence is linked to a clear understanding of the boundaries of an individual's own practice and more effective communication, which is critical to the facilitation and escalation of care needed during patient deterioration.[25]

"Simulation technology provides opportunities for learners to build skills and knowledge within a safe learning environment that protects patient safety, promotes active learning, presents specific and comparable patient situations, and supports error detection and response."[26] Modern simulators are technologically advanced with the capability to simulate hemodynamic monitoring, intubation, chest tube insertion, realistic lung sounds, cardiac arrhythmias, bleeding, seizures, pulses, and intravenous medication, and can respond to the learner's actions.

In addition to simulation being used in academia, there is a current trend to use simulation in the practice setting. Simulation training can be used in the so-called onboarding of new graduates and to identify patient safety issues such as medication administration safety; resuscitation training; team training; and events that are considered high risk, low volume. Preparing critical care nurses to care for the complex needs of unstable patients who have multiple tubes and lines, dressings, and several comorbidities is overwhelming. "Critical care orientations are designed to expose novice nurses to the intensive care environment and to prepare them to manage acute situations independently."[27]

Simulations that take place in the clinical area where the staff nurses work are referred to as in-situ training; the training can also occur in a simulation laboratory, set up to mimic a real unit. In-situ simulation may be planned during a typical work day or unannounced. Simulations that are unannounced provide a realism that provides the "contextual clues, practical difficulties, interruptions, and distractions of the real environment."[28] It is also essential for registered nurses to have sound communication skills. "Simulation training provides specific clinical learning experiences that place nurses in complex clinical situations requiring clinical judgment."[29] Ballangrud and colleagues[30] noted that simulation training for ICU nurses had "created awareness about clinical practice." Simulation for ICU nurses provides increased training in the areas of essential monitoring, such as pulmonary and cardiovascular values, intravenous medication administration, management of ventilatory status, level of consciousness, and code preparation.[27]

"Simulation technology provides opportunities for learners to build skills and knowledge within a safe learning environment that protects patient safety, promotes active learning, presents specific and comparable patient situations, and supports error detection and response."[26] The literature on the use of clinical simulation supports the use of simulation for nursing professional development to enhance knowledge and skills as well as confidence development.[6] Increased professional confidence has been associated with increased decision-making ability and decreased 30-day mortalities.[25] In addition, enhanced confidence is linked to a clear understanding of the boundaries of each clinician's own practice and enhanced communication. These outcomes are critical to the facilitation and escalation of care that are needed during patient deterioration.[25]

Applying the Algorithm

In designing an algorithm to be used in the care of patients with GI disorders in the ICU, recommendations from the National Institute of Health and Clinical Excellence were considered. These recommendations suggest that tools developed to augment care should consider care objectives, quantify individual risk factors, and identify criteria to recognize signs of deterioration using early warning scores.[31] Algorithms, much like decision trees or rubrics, help stimulate thought processes and may initiate communication among team members.[12] The development of the algorithm focused on risk factors for ICU patients with GI issues, anticipation of complications, and signs of deterioration that warrant escalation of care. Tanner's[11] clinical judgment model was then embedded into the algorithm to guide clinical judgment in the decision making (**Fig. 3**).

The first stage of model, noticing, is an interactive process that assumes that there is knowledge by the nurse of a clinical situation. This knowledge includes a contextual knowledge of the situation that directs the nurse in collecting clues about the patient's status and those changes that require attention. There is an expectation for the nurse to understand the critical connection between the GI system and organ failure risk. The clues collected should include current and related comorbidities that place the patient at high risk; these include but are not limited to sepsis, cardiac disorders,

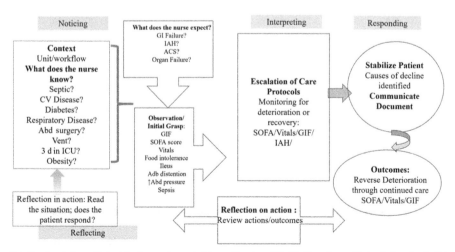

Fig. 3. Applying clinical judgment model to patients with GI disorders. Abd, abdominal; CV, cardiovascular, Vent, ventilator.

diabetes, and whether the patient has had abdominal surgery. From these data, the nurse draws inferences of the expectations of what could be occurring to the patient in this situation. Possibilities include GIF, IAH, ACS, or failure of 1 or more organs.

While moving through the stage of clinical judgment, the nurses perform additional assessments and data collection, which include the GIF score to assess GI function, the SOFA score, and vital sign changes based on the National Early Warning Score.[7] The algorithm gives suggestions for data combinations such as food intolerance, ileus, abdominal distention, increased abdominal pressure, and signs of sepsis that may point to GIF. Indications of high-risk patterns or additional organ failure (neurologic, respiratory, cardiovascular, and renal) are identified. Observation and assessment are followed by an analysis of why the patient is deteriorating and related factors precipitating or exacerbating the declining situation.

During the third phase, referred to as interpreting, actions are required in response to the analysis; the nurse is prompted in the algorithm to escalate care to stabilize the patient and prevent further deterioration. The nurse continues to assess the patient using the SOFA and GIF, and to assess vital signs, IAH and additional previously discussed data. Interventions are implemented based on care protocols and "the patient's response to the interventions may trigger further noticing and assessment, which refines the nurse's interpretation of the situation."[32]

The responding phase of the algorithm directs escalation of care, which includes active care processes and communication with care providers and other members of the health care team. The goal of this phase is to prevent further decline as patient outcomes are anticipated and a clearer understanding is obtained of why the patient is in a deteriorating situation. Care protocols are implemented addressing the source of GIF and related changes in another organ system.

Reflection is an essential aspect of the model and is intertwined throughout each stage of the process. Tanner[11] refers to this reflection as having 2 dimensions: reflection in action, which occurs throughout the process; and reflection on action, which occurs at the end of the model where outcomes are evaluated in conjunction with actions performed in the situation as well as a review of the process, considering the result to determine what caused the outcomes.[11] This stage is considered to be the final phase of Tanner's[11] model examining patient outcomes. At this point the reflection includes a review of the process, considering the result to determine what caused the outcomes. The actions performed are connected to outcomes to understand what occurred because of the actions.

The clinical judgment model, when embedded into this algorithm, could be used in simulation in various ways to prepare ICU nurses to identify and respond to patients with GI disorders in deteriorating situations. The remainder of this article discusses ways to use this algorithm using simulation.

Embedding an Algorithm into Simulation

The use of simulation, integrating an established theoretic framework for critical thinking, along with assessment tools such as the SOFA and the GIF scores embedded within an algorithm, can be powerful vehicles for preparing ICU nurses for decision making. Algorithms are frequently used in health care training in critical care settings; for example, the Advanced Cardiac Life Support algorithm. Some research has been performed on the use of algorithms in trauma medicine, and the results show consistency, a reduction in error rates, and also a reduction in the resuscitation time.[33] They provide a visual representation for decision making and reflect the complexity and possible choices that may occur during a patient situation.[34]

"Critical care orientations are designed to expose novice nurses to the intensive care environment and to prepare them to manage acute situations independently."[27] Simulation training can be used in the onboarding of new ICU nurses to help them in the identification of patient deterioration, resuscitation training, team training, and events that are considered high risk, low volume.

When planning training for staff nurses much can be learned from prelicensure training. Nurse educators in a practice should consider how ICU nurses process decision making using clinical reasoning and clinical judgment. There is much discussion in the literature about the differences between clinical judgment, clinical reasoning, and critical thinking; these terms are often used interchangeably. There is little argument with that both novice nurses and experienced nurses must rely on their ability to use these skills when caring for patients.

In 2006, Tanner[11] outlined a process by which nurses come to clinical decisions. Accurate and prompt clinical decision making can be key to early recognition of deterioration and ultimate rescue. Using the algorithm embedded with Tanner's[11] clinical judgment model can prompt clinical decision making that facilitates early recognition of deterioration and ultimate rescue. Nurse educators in the ICU can develop simulation training for acutely ill patients with GI conditions that includes moving the nurses through a scenario guided by Tanner's[11] model. Early recognition of patient deterioration is assessed in simulation through interpretation of observations collected through the SOFA and GIF scores, and management of care priorities is demonstrated during the simulation and reflected on during debriefing.

In the acute care setting, nurse educators can integrate the assessment algorithm during the development of the simulation activity. The educators should ensure that a needs assessment is completed first. This needs assessment can occur by tracking medical/nursing errors on a unit, by surveying the nurses about knowledge gaps, and through observation. Once the gap analysis has been performed and the objectives of the simulation have been developed, the nurse educator can work with the nurses on the unit to write the simulation case, using content experts to ensure validity of the content. Integrating the developed algorithm into the simulation to provide a roadmap for the staff is imperative. After piloting, the simulation event can be offered to the staff, or, depending on the knowledge gap, the event may be a required educational experience. As noted in Tanner's clinical judgment rubric and the developed algorithm, the reflection phase of the simulation event occurs both in action and on action; after the event, during the debriefing phase of simulation, further reflection regarding the simulation and care of the patients with GI disorders can occur. "Nurses care for patients with multifaceted issues; in the best interests of these patients, nurses often must consider a variety of conflicting and complex factors in choosing the best course of action."[12] Simulation, including the debriefing, is still a new tool used in acute care education but provides a safe place for nurses to develop their clinical judgment. Caring for patients with GI conditions in the ICU can be a daunting task; simulation and the implementation of the developed algorithm are tools that can be used to provide additional training and ultimately improve the care of patients with GI conditions.

SUMMARY

Nurses must be well prepared to make sound decisions that keep patients safe and prevent deterioration. The failure to recognize a patient's deterioration can lead to the patient not receiving accurate treatment and may increase mortality and morbidity.[8] The science of safety has matured to describe how communication breakdowns, diagnostic errors, poor judgment, and inadequate skill can directly result in patient harm and death.[3] Improved clinical outcomes for GI complications that lead to patient deterioration are imperative. Implementing simulation training is a tool that can be used to augment the training ICU nurses receive to examine the associated pertinent data and develop skill in the recognition of patient deterioration and the appropriate care responses. Simulation can be used to prepare ICU nurses to use tools to make accurate and safe patient care decisions.

Providing the nursing staff with adequate training when using such tools as algorithms can improve nurses' confidence and in turn the nurses can be more autonomous in their decision making. Simulation training integrated into this setting is becoming more popular in training staff nurses in the acute care setting. These "advanced, high-fidelity teaching methods that require participants to behave as they would in real life have been associated with improved learning and clinical outcomes."[35]

REFERENCES

1. Mapp ID, Davis LL, Krowchuk H. Prevention of unplanned intensive care unit admissions and hospital mortality by early warning systems. Dimens Crit Care Nurs 2013;32(6):300–9.
2. Valiee S, Peyrovi H, Nikbakht AK. Critical care nurses' perception of nursing error. Contemporary Nurse 2014;46(2):206–13.
3. Makary MA, Daniel M. Medical error—the third leading cause of death in the US. BMJ 2016;353:i2139.
4. Henriksen K, Dayton E, Keyes MA, et al. Chapter 5. Understanding adverse events: a human factors framework human factors — what is it? Saf Qual An Evidence-Based Handb Nurses. 2008:67–86.doi:NBK2666 [bookaccession].
5. Brown R, Rasmussen R, Baldwin I, et al. Design and implementation of a virtual world training simulation of ICU first hour handover processes. Aust Crit Care 2012;25(3):178–87.
6. Elder L. Simulation. J Nurses Prof Dev 2017;33(3):127–30.
7. Subbe CP, Welch JR. Failure to rescue: using rapid response systems to improve care of the deteriorating patient in hospital. Clin Risk 2013;19(1):6–11.
8. Garvey PK. Failure to rescue: The nurse's impact. MedSurg Nursing 2015;24(3):145–50.
9. Harvey EM, Echols SR, Clark R, et al. Comparison of two TeamSTEPPS® training methods on nurse failure-to-rescue performance. Clin Simul Nurs 2014. https://doi.org/10.1016/j.ecns.2013.08.006.
10. Perkins C, Kisiei M. Developing the recognition and response skills of student nurses. Br J Nurs 2013;22(12):715–25.
11. Tanner CA. Thinking like a nurse: a research-based model of clinical judgment in nursing. J Nurs Educ 2006;45(6):204–11.
12. Lasater K. Clinical judgment development: using simulation to create an assessment rubric. J Nurs Educ 2007;46(11):496–503.
13. Duhon JL. When organs fail one by one. RN 2006;69(5):44–9. Available at: www.rnweb.com.
14. Ferraris VA, Bolanos M, Martin JT, et al. Identification of patients with postoperative complications who are at risk for failure to rescue. JAMA Surg 2014;149(11):1103.
15. Vincent JL, Moreno R, Takala J, et al. The SOFA (Sepsis-related Organ Failure Assessment) score to describe organ dysfunction/failure. Intensive Care Med 1996;22(7):707–10. https://doi.org/10.1007/s001340050156.

16. Welton R, Faddoul B. Complications in bariatric patients: strategies to reduce failure to rescue. Bariatr Nurs Surg Patient Care 2009;4(1):53–7.
17. Vincent JL, Moreno R, Takala J, et al. The SOFA (sepsis-related organ failure assessment) score to describe organ dysfunction/failure. Intensive Care Med 1996;22(7):707–10.
18. Schorr CA, Zimmerman J. Updating and improving severity and prognostic measures. Crit Care Med 2015;43(7):1543–4.
19. Silvio AN. Application of the sequential organ failure assessment (SOFA) score to patients with cancer admitted to the intensive care unit. Am J Hosp Palliat Care 2009;26(5):341–6.
20. Blaser AR, Sarapuu S, Tamme K, et al. Expanded measurements of intra-abdominal pressure do not increase the detection rate of intra-abdominal hypertension. Crit Care Med 2014;42(2):378–86.
21. Lee RK. Intra-abdominal hypertension and abdominal compartment syndrome a comprehensive overview. Crit Care Nurse 2012;32(1):19–31.
22. Iyer D, Rastogi P, Aneman A, et al. Early screening to identify patients at risk of developing intra-abdominal hypertension and abdominal compartment syndrome. ACTA Anaesthesiol Scand 2014;58(10):1267–75. https://doi.org/10.1111/aas.12409.
23. Liang H, Daugherty EL, Taichman D, et al. Forced exhalation on the measurement of intraabdominal pressure. J Intensive Care Med 2008;23(4):268–74.
24. Ballangrud R, Persenius M, Hedelin B, et al. Exploring intensive care nurses' team performance in a simulation-based emergency situation, – expert raters' assessments versus self-assessments: an explorative study. BMC Nurs 2014;13(1):47.
25. Rao AD, Kumar A, McHugh M. Better nurse autonomy decreases the odds of 30-day mortality and failure to rescue. J Nurs Scholarsh 2017;49(1):73–9.
26. Liebrecht CM, Lieb MC. Incorporating quality and safety values into a CLABSI simulation experience. Nurs Forum 2016;52(2):118–23.
27. Stefanski RR, Rossler KL. Preparing the novice critical care nurse: a community-wide collaboration using the benefits of simulation. J Contin Educ Nurs 2009;40(10):443–51, 453.
28. Walker ST, Sevdalis N, McKay A, et al. Unannounced in situ simulations: integrating training and clinical practice. BMJ Qual Saf 2013;22(6):453–8.
29. Martin MG, Keller LA, Long TL, et al. High-fidelity simulation effect on nurses' identification of deteriorating pediatric patients. Clin Simul Nurs 2016;12(6):228–39.
30. Ballangrud R, Hall-Lord ML, Persenius M, et al. Intensive care nurses' perceptions of simulation-based team training for building patient safety in intensive care: a descriptive qualitative study. Intensive Crit Care Nurs 2014;30(4):179–87.
31. Lavoie P, Pepin J, Cossette S. Development of a post-simulation debriefing intervention to prepare nurses and nursing students to care for deteriorating patients. Nurse Educ Pract 2015;15(3):181–91.
32. Schoessler M. Tanner's model of clinical judgment applied to preceptorship: part 1. J Nurses Prof Dev 2013;29(5):274–5.
33. Lee GA, Murray A, Bushnell R, et al. Challenges developing evidence-based algorithms for the trauma reception and resuscitation project. Int Emerg Nurs 2013;21(2):129–35.
34. Bartlett JL. A simulation template for a new simulation program. Clin Simul Nurs 2015;11(11):479–81.
35. Jansson MM, Syrjala HP, Ohtonen PP, et al. Randomized, controlled trial of the effectiveness of simulation education: a 24-month follow-up study in a clinical setting. Am J Infect Control 2016;44(4):387–93.

Evidence-Based Practice in the Treatment for Antibiotic-Associated Diarrhea in the Intensive Care Unit

Robin Squellati, PhD, APRN-C*

KEYWORDS

- Diarrhea • Antibiotic • *Clostridium difficile* • Probiotics • Spores • Vancomycin

KEY POINTS

- The use of antibiotics leads to diarrhea.
- *Clostridium difficile* infection (CDI) is a serious hospital-acquired infection.
- Contact precautions need to begin when diarrhea is identified.
- Vancomycin is used to treat CDI.

Antibiotic-associated diarrhea (AAD) is a common occurrence in intensive care units (ICU) across the United States. Antibiotics can disrupt the normal gut microbiota and cause AAD.[1] Some patients who have AAD develop *Clostridium difficile* colonization or infection. More than 500,000 people were known to contract *C difficile* infections (CDI) while hospitalized in 2011, and the trend for CDIs is increasing.[2] The Centers for Disease Control and Prevention are tracking CDI through the Emerging Infections Program, in which many states and academic health centers are participating. Of the one-half million persons who contracted *C difficile* in 2011, 29,000 died.[2] CDI costs the United States more than 4.8. billion dollars per year, just for acute care facilities.[3] The additional acute care costs were from longer hospitalizations, contact isolation, laboratory fees, and antibiotics. These costs are expected to double over the next 4 decades because the population over age 65 is increasing.[4] Elderly patients in surgical units and ICU are the most susceptible to CDI.[5] Many medications, including antibiotics, list diarrhea among the side effects. CDI is the number one cause of nosocomial infections.[6] The purpose of this article is to inform nurses about AAD, describe the antibiotics

---

The author has no financial interests, affiliations, or conflicts of interest that relate to the publication of this material.

MSN SP Program, Walden University, Minneapolis, MN, USA

* 3155 Tedesco Court, Sparks, NV 89434.

E-mail address: robin.squellati@mail.waldenu.edu

that are more likely to lead to both AAD and CDI, and to explore the role of probiotics in prevention of AAD. Last, what ICU nurses can do to decrease the incidence of AAD and CDI is discussed.

WHO IS PRONE TO ANTIBIOTIC-ASSOCIATED DIARRHEA AND WHY?

AAD affects 25% to 30% of the people taking antibiotics.[6] AAD is usually defined as 3 loose stools in a 24-hour period while on antibiotics or after completing the course of antibiotics.[1,7,8] If the patient has 3 episodes of unformed stool in 24 hours, testing for CDI and consideration to stop or change antibiotics is recommended.[2] One reason for AAD is that broad-spectrum antibiotics disrupt the normal interaction of the microbiota and host, leading to diarrhea.[8] Some patients are more likely to develop AAD and require special consideration when beginning a new antibiotic.

Patients over the age of 65, those on proton pump inhibitors (PPI), or those having a prior hospitalization, especially within the previous 3 months, are prone to AAD.[2,9,10] Also, patients on chemotherapy, with immunocompromised conditions, or having diabetes are more likely to develop AAD.[11] Lin and colleagues[11] looked at 486 patients, where 86 (17.8%) developed colonization with C difficile, and found that diabetes mellitus, piperacillin–tazobactam, or those on a protein pump inhibitors had a higher rate of C difficile–associated diarrhea (CDAD). There were no statistical differences between body mass index or gender for those who acquire AAD and those who do not develop AAD.[11] Besides underlying conditions, antibiotics, and age, PPIs may contribute to CDAD.

Nurses are well aware that antibiotics may lead to diarrhea, but Gordon and colleagues[12] questioned if receiving high-risk antibiotics and being on a PPI caused greater risk of AAD. With 3513 patients on high-risk antibiotics and a PPI, and 6149 who were on high-risk antibiotics, but not a PPI, 111 total patients were positive for CDI. The conclusion was that using high-risk antibiotics and a PPI had a significantly higher rate of CDI. Therefore, avoidance of PPIs for patients in the ICU when possible could decrease the morbidity of CDI. Abdelfatah and colleagues[13] performed a retrospective study of 3020 patients who were positive for CDI. This study found that glucocorticoids, use of PPIs, and end-stage renal disease place patients at risk for recurrent CDI.[13] Faleck and colleagues[14] studied 18,134 ICU patient records to determine predictive factors for CDI. The question was whether patients in the ICU were different from other patients, with respect to causes of CDI.[14] The results showed that, like other studies, antibiotics were the strongest predictive factor for CDI. However, unlike other studies, there was not an increased risk of CDI for those on a PPI. Finally, a large international study was done with more than 3 million patients, and 54,957 patients selected for review.[15] The results showed an association between PPIs and CDI in this group. Like with antibiotics, the PPI must be considered a risk factor for hospitalized, high-risk patients.

Also, infectious diarrhea may be caused by the norovirus, Clostridium perfringens, Klebsiella oxytoca, and Bacteroides fragilis. B fragilis is a community-acquired diarrhea-causing organism, but is rarely a cause of nosocomial diarrhea. Testing for these organisms and other causes of diarrhea is limited.[8] K oxytoca creates a toxin that impedes DNA syntheses, and causes bloody diarrhea.[8] C perfringens also causes bloody diarrhea, which usually resolves in 24 hours without treatment.[1] Staphylococcus aureus is a rare cause of AAD.[1] CDI causes diarrhea, cramping, and severe abdominal pain, and begins 48 to 72 hours after introduction of the organism.[1] The patient may have 10 to 15 loose stools per day, which means that a significant amount of fluids and electrolytes are lost. Besides bacteria, AAD may also result from *Candida*, which may require nystatin to treat.[5] Not only do organisms cause diarrhea, but underlying health conditions may lead to diarrhea.

Noninfectious diarrhea may be caused by several disease conditions like inflammatory bowel disease, irritable bowel syndrome, and diabetic enteropathy, which can lead to diarrhea. Also, substance abuse withdrawal causes diarrhea.[8] Patients hospitalized for a short duration have less than a 5% chance of developing diarrhea in the hospital. The medical history, and consideration of all medications, a change of diet, and travel outside the country are important to understanding the cause of the diarrhea. Most hospitalized patients with diarrhea have a noninfectious etiology. Still, up to one-third of AAD is from *C difficile*.[6] With AAD, it is important to test for *C difficile*, because *C difficile* can be deadly, and needs to be treated as soon as possible. **Table 1** depicts the frequency of some causes of AAD.

Prolonged hospitalization is another risk factor.[9] Patients in the ICU may have a longer duration of stay. In the ICU, ventilator-acquired pneumonia (VAP) is a common reason for antibiotic use.[16] Hellyer and colleagues[16] conducted a randomized controlled trial on using bronchoalveolar lavage for patients who were diagnosed

Table 1
Relative frequency of *Clostridium difficile* and other causes of nosocomial diarrhea in high-risk patient subgroups

	Antibiotics	Intensive Care	Chemotherapy	SOT	HSCT
Diarrhea (total)[a]	5%–25%	≥15%–40%	20%–80%	7%–27%	43%–79%
Infectious (% of total)[b]	10%–30%	10%–30%[c]	≤20%[d]	17%–20%	6%–19%
C difficile[b]	10%–25%	10%–25%[c]	10%–14%	5%–10%	1%–20%
Other toxigenic bacteria[b,e]	1%–8%	1%–8%[c]	Unknown	Unknown	Unknown
Norovirus and other viruses[b]	Unknown	Unknown	Unknown	Unknown	8%[f]
Opportunistic infections (cytomegalovirus)[b]	N/S	N/S	N/S	≤5%	<5%
Noninfectious (% of total)[g]	70%–90%	70%–90%[c]	≥80%[d]	80%–83%	81%–94%

Abbreviations: HSCT, hematopoietic stem cell transplant; N/S, not significant; SOT, solid organ transplant.
[a] Proportion of patients developing diarrhea in each risk group.
[b] Proportion of total diarrheal episodes in risk group attributable to an infectious cause or individual infectious agent.
[c] Data not available for intensive care population. Specified percentages are for antibiotic-associated diarrhea.
[d] Estimated percentage; data not available for chemotherapy patients.
[e] Antibiotic-associated: *Clostridium perfringens*, *Klebsiella oxytoca*, and *Staphylococcus aureus*.
[f] Most often adenovirus, astrovirus, or rotavirus; likely includes a mix of nosocomial and community infections.
[g] Proportion of total diarrheal episodes with no infectious cause identified.
From Polage C, Solnick J, Cohen S. Nosocomial diarrhea: evaluation and treatment of causes other than Clostridium difficile. Clin Infect Dis 2012;55(7):986; with permission.

with VAP. Biomarkers were used to determine the need for antibiotic use. There were 210 patients in the study. The results of using biomarkers were rapid discontinuation of antibiotics. VAP bundles, including raising the head of bed, daily assessment of readiness to extubate, use of subglottic secretion drainage, and avoidance of scheduled ventilator circuit changes was recommended.[17] The use of oral chlorhexidine was not recommended, owing to increased mortality in some patients.[17] Antibiotic stewardship is needed.

WHY DO ANTIBIOTICS CAUSE DIARRHEA, AND WHICH ANTIBIOTICS ARE PRONE TO CAUSING DIARRHEA?

About 50% of hospitalized patients receive an antibiotic.[2] Of patients who develop CDI, 99% were on an antibiotic within 90 days before the CDI diagnosis.[18] A study by Srigley and colleagues[18] found that the antibiotics prescribed for pneumonia were the most common reason for antibiotic use, and 28.4% did not meet the diagnostic criteria for pneumonia. The second most common use of hospital antibiotics was for urinary tract infections, but 75% of these cases did not need antibiotics. Perioperative antibiotic prophylaxis was found to be inappropriate in 83% of the cases. Using an infectious disease team for pneumonia, UTIs, and perioperative cases could help to guide antibiotic stewardship.

Antibiotics lead to AAD for a few reasons. One is that the normal flora of the gut has been disrupted, leading to nondigested carbohydrates.[1] This condition causes osmotic diarrhea. Also, bile salts are not absorbed in the small bowel, and become bile acids by bacteria in the colon, causing secretory diarrhea.[1] A few of the antibiotics associated with AAD and CDAD are clindamycin, cephalosporins, and fluoroquinolones.[19] McDonald and colleagues[19] found that 77% of patients with CDI received at least 1 dose of an unnecessary antibiotic.

In a study by Haran and colleagues,[20] 275 patients who received antibiotics in the emergency department developed AAD. About 20% of the patients developed AAD and 4 were positive for CDI. The most common medication causing AAD was clindamycin, and the one least likely to cause diarrhea was vancomycin. Likewise, the ICU has challenges with antibiotics.

Antibiotic use in the ICU may be prolonged or may be prescribed when antibiotics are not indicated.[21] Either situation could lead to AAD. Biomarkers, such as procalcitonin, were studied to help clinicians determine if stopping an antibiotic is warranted. Albrich and Harbarth[21] looked at randomized controlled trials, and found that, in severe sepsis or septic shock, procalcitonin could be used as a biomarker, but in other cases, biomarkers did not provide the guidance for initiating or stopping antibiotics.

Ampicillin causes AAD 5% to 10% of the time, cefixime causes diarrhea 15% to 20% of the time, and amoxicillin-clavulate causes AAD 10% to 25% of the time. Sarma and colleagues[22] found that reducing the use of cephalosporins and fluoroquinolones also reduced the incidence of CDI. Diarrhea and CDI began increasing as the use of clindamycin and penicillins increased.[5] Broad-spectrum antibiotics and concomitant antibiotics tend to lead to CDAD.[23]

Aminoglycosides, sulfonamides, macrolides, tetracycline, and vancomycin are the best antibiotics to use to avoid AAD and CDAD. Vancomycin given orally as a treatment for CDI is advantageous owing to the body's inability to fully absorb the medication, leaving vancomycin in the colon to fight the infection. Electrolyte replacement must also be considered owing to the loss of fluids with AAD.[8] Surgical treatment is sometimes necessary with CDI, where a subtotal colectomy or diverting loop ileostomy with colonic lavage is used.[5] **Table 2** clarifies the antibiotics that most often lead to CDI.

Table 2
Antibiotic groups that may predispose to C difficile infection

Commonly	Occasionally	Seldom
Fluoroquinolones	Macrolides	Aminoglycosides
Clindamycin	Trimethoprim	Tetracyclines
Penicillins	Sulfonamides	Chloramphenicol
Cephalosporins		Metronidazole
		Vancomycin

From Kazanowski M, Smolarek S, Kinnarney F, et al. Clostridium difficile: epidemiology, diagnostic and therapeutic possibilities-a systematic review. Tech Coloproctol 2012;18(3):225; with permission.

CLOSTRIDIUM DIFFICILE INFECTIONS

C difficile is a gram-positive, anaerobic bacillus, which is found in the environment, most commonly in soil.[5] *C difficile* was first identified in 1935, and was given the name *difficile*, a Latin word for difficult, because *C difficile* was difficult to isolate, and had a slow growth phase during culture. Still today, a rapid, reliable laboratory test is not readily available.[24] Stool cultures frequently give false-positive results, so a toxigenic culture is needed. However, most laboratories are not equipped for anaerobic cultures, and culture results take 48 to 96 hours.[2] Molecular testing for *C difficile* with an accurate assay test as early possible helps to begin treatment earlier, and may decrease morbidity. The polymerase chain reaction ribotyping has a specificity of up to 97%. Antigen testing for *C difficile* can be resulted in less than 1 hour. This test is nonspecific, which means another confirmatory test is needed, but if positive, and the patient had risk factors for CDI (**Table 3**), precautions and treatment could be taken sooner. The enzyme immunoassays can test for toxins A and B, or both, and can offer results in 1 day, but have the disadvantage of less sensitivity.[2] The nucleic acid amplification test is a newer, more sensitive test, but is slow to be adopted by laboratories across the United States.[3] Reliable testing is needed, because *C difficile* is such a serious disease, and the cost of testing equipment could be offset by obtaining accurate results sooner.

C difficile is the major cause of death in patients with inflammatory bowel disease.[5] Why focus on CDI versus other causes of diarrhea? About 10% of patients with CDI will die.[6] The organism is highly contagious. Also, patients incur a longer duration of

Table 3
Reported risk factors for *Clostridium difficile* infection

Measures	Findings
Reported risk factors	Hospitalization or long duration of stay
	Antimicrobial use, although some CA-CDI cases found to have no recent antibiotic exposure
	Older age
	CA-CDI cases younger than HO-HCFA-CDI cases
	Comorbidity
	PPIs and H2 antagonists

Abbreviations: CA, community-associated; CDI, *clostridium difficile* infection; HCFA, health care facility-associated; HO, health care facility onset; PPI, proton pump inhibitor.
From Evans C, Safdar N. Current trends in the epidemiology and outcomes of Clostridium difficile infection. Clin Infect Dis 2015;60(Suppl 2):S67; with permission.

hospital stay (average, 6.4 days), which costs between $10,000 and $15,000 per patient. Overall, in the United States, the cost of CDI is $3.2 billion.[23] This is a difficult bacteria owing to *C difficile*–forming spores, which remain on inanimate surfaces.[9] Patients with a leukocyte count, fever, elevated creatinine, and albumin of less than 2.5 mg/dL should be admitted to the ICU.[5] ICU nurses need to be aware of the seriousness of CDI. **Table 4** shows the mortality and costs of CDI.

The spore form of CDI is resistant to regular cleaning and requires using sporicidal agents.[23] The spores are not affected by alcohol-based hand sanitizers, or usual environmental cleaning agents.[2,23] Even handwashing may not eliminate *C difficile*. Therefore, gloves are required. Also, the spores survive on inanimate objects and are ingested.[7] *C difficile* must be identified as soon as possible to begin precautions to keep health care staff from spreading the organism.

The number of cases of CDI is continually increasing.[9] The most common type of CDI was found to be the North American pulsed-field gel electrophoresis type 1 (NAP1) strain when 15,461 cases of CDI were reviewed in a large, longitudinal study across the United States.[3] CDI is the most common hospital-acquired infection.[9,25] The organism causes diarrhea, pseudomembranous colitis, toxic megacolon, colonic perforation, and death.[9] A toxin, B toxin, and binary toxin are associated with hospital-acquired *C difficile*.[26] CDI strain BI is an especially severe strain of CDI.[27] Once A toxin gets into the cell, increased intestinal permeability and fluid secretion result. B toxin results in colonic inflammation.[28] CDI causes 15% to 25% of AAD.[26] Either toxin has a high mortality rate, which can be up to 15%.

From a systematic review, Kazanowski and colleagues[5] found also that *C difficile* is responsible for outbreaks of diarrhea in hospitals. As CDI progresses, colitis may occur, which is manifested by fever, leukocytosis, a positive fecal occult blood test, and abdominal guarding.[5] The next stage is pseudomembranous colitis, in which a yellow plaque is observed during colonoscopy. Once cured from pseudomembranous colitis, there is still a 10% to 25% recurrence rate, and the reinfection is usually more severe.[5] An effective treatment for CDI is needed.

Petrella and colleagues[27] studied fidaxomicin compared with vancomycin to determine which antibiotic was most effective. There were 999 patients in the study and 86.6% had cure rates. CDI was cured at a rate of 94.3%. The use of fidaxomicin was comparable with using vancomycin. Other toxic strains are NAP1 and 027.[10] NAP1 and 027 have mobile and mosaic genomes, which makes them more drug resistant.[28]

Table 4	
***Clostridium difficile* infection outcomes**	
Measures	**Findings**
CDI outcomes	
Recurrence	20%–30%
Colectomy	8.7 per 1000 CDI cases
Mortality	14,000 deaths per year
	90% of CDI deaths are in elderly
Costs	$2454–$29,000 per episode
	$4.8 billion in excess costs to US acute care facilities
Duration of stay (d)	2.7–21.3

From Evans C, Safdar N. Current trends in the epidemiology and outcomes of Clostridium difficile infection. Clin Infect Dis Clin Infect Dis 2015;60(Suppl 2):S67; with permission.

Should patients who are CDI carriers, but have no symptoms, be isolated? Grigoras and colleagues[25] looked at testing patients for CDI upon admission, and then isolating the patient if a positive CDI result was obtained. On admission 6.18 of 1000 patients had CDI, but upon discharge the rate of CDI was 9.72 in 1000 patients. Screening and isolation led to a 36.2% reduction in CDI upon discharge. Also, Grigoras and colleagues[25] simulated an antimicrobial stewardship program which reduced the CDI rate to 2.35 in 1000 admissions. Blixt and colleagues[29] found that, in a large study of 4508 patients, C difficile carriers could contribute to nosocomial CDI. An antimicrobial stewardship bundle included screening upon admission, and if positive for CDI, the patient was placed on contact precautions for the duration of the hospitalization.

In a similar study, Zacharioudakis and colleagues[10] theorized that colonization with C difficile leads to greater risk of CDI. Zacharioudakis and colleagues[10] reviewed 19 studies (8725 patients) and found that 8% of patients are carriers of C difficile. These patients have a 6 times greater risk of CDI. C difficile carriers should be identified upon admission to reduce the chances of CDI and to prevent transmission to other patients.[10] Colonized patients are asymptomatic, but can still transmit CDI.[5] In ICUs, the carrier rate can be as high as 20% to 50%.[5] However, others claim it is usually unnecessary to test for C difficile in the absence of symptoms.[7] Estimates of the number of C difficile–colonized people may be low, giving a false sense of security. The actual numbers that have been reported are 0% to 15% for healthy adults, and 6% to 15% for the elderly.[7]

In another study, Delate and colleagues[30] reviewed community-associated CDI and nosocomial CDI in 1201 patients. Patients with nosocomial CDI were older, more likely to have a CDI recurrence, and more likely to die. The conclusion was that patients who had community-associated CDI were much different from those with nosocomial CDI. However, this study did not look at the type of CDI toxins.[30] Lessa and colleagues[3] found that 46% of CDI cases were community-associated CDI, and of those 82% had visited a clinic within 12-week before being diagnosed with a CDI. Søes and colleagues[26] found that community-associated CDI was 30%.

Animals have been thought to carry C difficile. Stone and colleagues[31] found that pet dogs carry the same pathogenic strain of C difficile as found in humans. Stone and colleagues[31] concluded that pet dogs are a potential source of community acquired C difficile. However, McDonald and colleagues[19] reported that 94% of CDI was associated with health care exposure.

ARE PROBIOTICS HELPFUL IN PREVENTING ANTIBIOTIC-ASSOCIATED DIARRHEA?

C difficile bacteria are able to colonize the gastrointestinal tract when the normal flora are altered by antibiotics.[5] Therefore, the first step in treatment is to stop the antibiotic. In about 20% of patients, CDI will resolve in 2 days with just stopping the antibiotic.[2] Probiotics are sometimes used along with antibiotics, because probiotics may help to counteract the negative effect of antibiotics on the gastrointestinal flora.[32] Probiotics are live microorganisms aimed at restoring the gut microbiota.[33] Probiotics help to reduce colonization of C difficile by adhering to the epithelial and mucosal membranes.[34] However, are there any adverse reactions from taking probiotics?

Johnston and colleagues[32] performed a systematic review and metaanalysis of 20 trials with 3818 patients to determine if probiotics were effective to prevent CDAD. They found that moderate quality evidence shows that probiotics reduce the chance of CDAD to a large extent, and with only a small percentage of adverse reactions. The probiotics used in the studies were Bifidobacterium, Lactobacillus, Saccharomyces, and Streptococcus.[32] Szajewska and Kołodziej[35] performed a systematic review of

21 randomized controlled trials (4780 participants) found that AAD can be prevented with *Saccharomyces boulardii*, a probiotic. Another double-blind, randomized controlled trial evaluated the probiotic VSL#3 (*Bifidobacterium* and *Lactobacillus*) versus placebo twice daily for the duration of the antibiotic plus 7 days.[36] The conclusion was that average-risk patients had a significant reduction in ADD with VSL#3, but no cases of CDAD were reported in either group. Therefore, a dilemma is understanding which probiotics are best, and the dosage and frequency of the probiotic.

A large randomized controlled trial (n = 2981) to study the effects of probiotics on AAD was done in the UK.[37] This study, PLACIDE (Lactobacilli and Bifidobacteria in the prevention of antibiotic-associated diarrhoea and Clostridium difficile diarrhoea in older inpatients), used was 2 strains of *Lactobacillus acidophilus* and 2 strains of *Bifidobacterium*. The results were that AAD and CDI were not decreased in the probiotic group compared with the placebo group. This study was significant, because it was prospective, large, and a randomized controlled trial. Still, probiotics are considered a low-cost method to try to reduce AAD. In contrast with the PLACIDE study, another metaanalysis of 82 randomized controlled trials showed that probiotics did reduce AAD.[33]

Health Canada suggests using probiotics in the prevention of CDAD.[23] Canada used 50 billion colony-forming units of *L acidophilus* and *Lactobacillus casei*. Weed[38] reviewed 31 randomized controlled trials, including 4492 patients, and found the results showed that probiotics reduced AAD. However, probiotics were not shown to prevent CDI. Still, to reduce AAD, without significant adverse reactions, would make probiotics beneficial. A Cochrane review of 23 randomized controlled trials and 4213 patients found moderate quality evidence that probiotics are safe and effective.[39] Videlock and Cremonini[40] conducted a metaanalysis that included 34 studies (4138 patients) who were given probiotics versus a placebo. The probiotics were used during and after the use of an antibiotic. The results showed a preventive effect of the probiotics, regardless of the probiotic used, the population, or the duration of the probiotic. Wright and colleagues[41] used a double-blinded randomized controlled trial to evaluate the effectiveness of *L casei*, Shriota strain versus placebo to prevent AAD. There was no statistical difference between the probiotic group and the placebo group, but the sample size was only 87 patients. Xie and colleagues[34] performed a systematic review of 6 randomized controlled trials, 3562 patients, receiving *Lactobacillus*, *Bifidobacterium*, *Saccharomyces*, *Streptococcus*, *Enterococcus*, and *Bacillus*. Only 1 trial with *Bacillus licheniformis* was effective in the prevention of AAD. Also, there is not a known best type or combination of probiotics, amount, frequency, or duration to prevent AAD.

Probiotics should not be used in the ICU, owing to some patients having an adverse reaction, while already compromised owing to the patient's underlying condition.[6] However, Varughese and colleagues[6] found probiotics to be safe and well-tolerated, except in cases of probiotic bacteremia, which may occur in patients with cardiac valvular disease, short gut syndrome, and probiotics administered via the jejunostomy tube. Probiotics cannot be recommended routinely with the current evidence.[6] So, antibiotic stewardship, using PPIs only when absolutely necessary, and preventing health care-acquired infections would be the best actions to prevent AAD.

WHAT CAN NURSES DO TO PREVENT *CLOSTRIDIUM DIFFICILE* INFECTIONS?

As with most complex problems, to decrease CDIs, several measures are required. The European Center for Disease Prevention and the Society for Healthcare Epidemiology of America/Infectious Diseases Society of America recommended guidelines to control the transmission of CDI.[23] Among the guidelines were staff education, antibiotic stewardship, reduction of risk factors, the use of probiotics, hand hygiene, specific CDI environmental cleaning, medical equipment disinfection, early detection of CDI, and isolation techniques. Bernard and Little[42] researched environmental cleaning and found that even with bleach cleaning, patients were still acquiring CDI. However, after an ultraviolet disinfection system was added to the current bundle of CDI precautions, CDI decreased by 41%.[42]

Even though diarrhea may be caused from a noninfectious etiology, it is still recommended to use contact precautions as soon as possible.[2] Additionally, the patient will still shed *C difficile* for several days after the diarrhea has stopped. Therefore, contact isolation needs to continue for several days, and if the patient is transferred, the new facility needs to be aware.[2] Because antibiotic stewardship is a good method to decrease CDI, a study looked at decision making for the use of antibiotics.[43] ICUs battle infections daily, and often antibiotics are started without adequate objective evidence, which leads to AAD. Information technology could be used to help with antibiotic decision making. As soon as the culture and sensitivity results are available, check to be certain the antibiotic being used is right for the organism.[2] **Fig. 1** offers an algorithm to decide if simple standard preventive measures or probiotics should be used.

As always, nurses can decrease the risk of an infection through proper hand washing, wearing gloves, and using contact precautions. Nurses need to prevent catheter-associated infections and VAP by following best practices. An infection leads to antibiotic use.[23] Nurses need to alert physicians if the patient is on a PPI. Decreasing the risk of AAD and an infection is possible.

Withholding PPIs during antibiotic therapy should be considered.[22] Also, restrict the use of cephalosporins and fluoroquinolones. Use ultraviolet methods for terminal cleaning and a sporicidal agent for daily cleaning. Perform a root cause analysis for

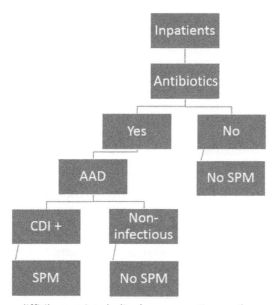

Fig. 1. *Clostridium difficile*–associated diarrhea prevention pathway. AAD, antibiotic-associated diarrhea; CDI, *C difficile* infection; SPM, standard preventive measures. (*Adapted from* Goldstein E, Johnson S, Low D, et al. Pathway to prevention of nosocomial clostridium difficile infection. Clin Infect Dis 2015;60 Suppl 2:S156; with permission.)

all CDI cases. By following these precautions, reduction of CDI cases went from 208 to 72 over a period of 2 years at 9 different hospitals.[22]

To prevent recurrence of CDI, oral vancomycin was tapered over 6 weeks. Rifaximin may also be used over 2 weeks to reduce the recurrence of *C difficile*.[5] Another approach is to give metronidazole to patients receiving broad-spectrum antibiotics.[44] Rodriguez and colleagues[44] retrospectively reviewed 12,026 patient records, and found that the incidence of CDAD was lower (1.4% compared with 6.5%) in patients who received metronidazole. This was an 80% decrease for a low cost. Patients could be identified for risk, and then evaluated to determine if the patient should receive metronidazole.

People with recurrent CDI may also try fecal microbiota transplantation, which has been approved by the American College of Gastroenterology and the Infectious Diseases Society of America.[28] Patients in the ICU may choose this as an adjunct therapy, because it is inexpensive, and can restore the gut microbiota. Recurrent cases have multiple recurrences in 50% of the cases, and often require fecal microbiota transplantation.[45] The 2 preferred methods of fecal microbiota transplantation are via colonoscopy or by enema, and both are from 81% to 100% effective.[28]

New antibiotics are needed; over time, organisms can become resistant to the current antibiotics. A new antibiotic to treat CDI, cadazolid, seems promising. Cadazolid is a combination of oxazolidinone and quinolone, with less CDI recurrence and less intestinal dysbiosis.[46] Currently, some strains of CDI are resistant to metronidazole, leaving only vancomycin to treat CDI.[46]

SUMMARY

The economic, social, and individual costs of AAD have become a huge burden on our country. Patients are hospitalized with an expectation that their health condition will be treated, and do not expect to develop a health care-acquired infection. There are several best practices that can be followed to prevent infections, such as following protocol for early removal of catheters, VAP bundles, and surgical site infection prevention. Patients who are older, on PPIs, or have immunocompromised conditions are at greater risk. Also, those who are prescribed broad-spectrum antibiotics or concomitant antibiotics are at great risk of AAD. A few of these antibiotics include clindamycin, cephalosporins, and fluoroquinolones. Many of these antibiotics may not even be necessary.[18] Antibiotic stewardship is important to decrease the chance of CDI, which can result in an increased duration of hospitalization, colitis, pseudomembranous colitis, toxic megacolon, or even death.[9] Unfortunately, the trend for CDI is increasing, and is expected to continue the trend as more Baby Boomers reach the age of 65.[2] Probiotics have been suggested as a means to decrease AAD and CDI, and several studies have showed the effectiveness of probiotics.[32,34,35] However, the large PLACIDE study did not show similar results.[37] So, nurses must rely on better hand hygiene, using contact precautions for those with AAD, environmental cleaning with a sporicidal solution, ensuring antibiotic stewardship, and decreased use of PPIs. Testing for CDI must be done with a reliable test as soon as possible. ICU nurses can stop AAD and CDI, and must do so to make hospitals a safe place for patients.

REFERENCES

1. Varughese C, Vakil N, Phillips K. Antibiotic-associated diarrhea: a refresher on causes and possible prevention with probiotics - continuing education article. J Pharm Pract 2013;(5):476.

2. Healthcare-associated infections – *Clostridium difficile* infection. Centers for Disease Control and Prevention. 2017. Available at: https://www.cdc.gov/hai/organisms/cdiff/cdiff_infect.html. Accessed March 1, 2017.

3. Lessa F, Yi M, McDonald L, et al. Burden of clostridium difficile infection in the United States. N Engl J Med 2015;(9):825.

4. Hübner C, Hübner N, Flessa S, et al. Cost analysis of hospitalized Clostridium difficile-associated diarrhea (CDAD). GMS Hyg Infect Control 2015;10:Doc13.

5. Kazanowski M, Smolarek S, Kinnarney F, et al. Clostridium difficile: epidemiology, diagnostic and therapeutic possibilities-a systematic review. Tech Coloproctol 2014;18(3):223–32.

6. Johnson DA. Probiotics: help or harm in antibiotic-associated diarrhea? 2014. Available at: http://www.medscape.com/viewarticle/830002. Accessed March 1, 2017.

7. Furuya-Kanamori L, Marquess J, Clements A, et al. Asymptomatic Clostridium difficile colonization: epidemiology and clinical implications. BMC Infect Dis 2015;15:516.

8. Polage C, Solnick J, Cohen S. Nosocomial diarrhea: evaluation and treatment of causes other than Clostridium difficile. Clin Infect Dis 2012;55(7):982–9.

9. Evans C, Safdar N. Current trends in the epidemiology and outcomes of Clostridium difficile infection. Clin Infect Dis 2015;(10):66.

10. Zacharioudakis I, Zervou F, Pliakos E, et al. Colonization with toxinogenic C. difficile upon hospital admission, and risk of infection: a systematic review and meta-analysis. Am J Gastroenterol 2015;110(3):381–90.

11. Lin HJ, Hung YP, Liu HC, et al. Risk factors for Clostridium difficile-associated diarrhea among hospitalized adults with fecal toxigenic C. difficile colonization. J Microbiol Immunol Infect 2015;48(2):183–9.

12. Gordon D, Young L, Reddy S, et al. Incidence of Clostridium difficile infection in patients receiving high-risk antibiotics with or without a proton pump inhibitor. J Hosp Infect 2016;92(2):173–7.

13. Abdelfatah M, Nayfe R, Kandil H, et al. Factors predicting recurrence of Clostridium difficile infection (CDI) in hospitalized patients: retrospective study of more than 2000 patients. J Investig Med 2015;63(5):747–51.

14. Faleck DM, Salmasian H, Furuya EY, et al. Proton pump inhibitors do not increase risk for Clostridium difficile infection in the intensive care unit. Am J Gastroenterol 2016;111(11):1641–8.

15. Roughead EE, Chan EW, Choi N, et al. Proton pump inhibitors and risk of Clostridium difficile infection: a multi-country study using sequence symmetry analysis. Expert Opin Drug Saf 2016;15(12):1589–95.

16. Hellyer T, Anderson N, Simpson A, et al. Effectiveness of biomarker-based exclusion of ventilator-acquired pneumonia to reduce antibiotic use (VAPrapid-2): study protocol for a randomised controlled trial. Trials 2016;17(1):318.

17. Hellyer T, Ewan V, Wilson P, et al. The Intensive Care Society recommended bundle of interventions for the prevention of ventilator-associated pneumonia. J Intensive Care Soc 2016;17(3):238.

18. Srigley J, Brooks A, Sung M, et al. Inappropriate use of antibiotics and Clostridium difficile infection. Am J Infect Control 2013;41(11):1116–8.

19. McDonald LC, Lessa F, Sievert D, et al. Vital signs: preventing Clostridium difficile infections. MMWR Morb Mortal Wkly Rep 2012;61(9):157–62.

20. Haran J, Hayward G, Boyer E, et al. Factors influencing the development of antibiotic associated diarrhea in ED patients discharged home: risk of administering IV antibiotics. Am J Emerg Med 2014;32(10):1195–9.

21. Albrich W, Harbarth S. Pros and cons of using biomarkers versus clinical decisions in start and stop decisions for antibiotics in the critical care setting. Intensive Care Med 2015;(10):1739.

22. Sarma J, Marshall B, Cleeve V, et al. Effects of fluoroquinolone restriction (from 2007 to 2012) on resistance in Enterobacteriaceae: interrupted time-series analysis. J Hosp Infect 2015;91(1):68–73.

23. Goldstein E, Johnson S, Low D, et al. Pathway to prevention of nosocomial Clostridium difficile infection. Clin Infect Dis 2015;60(Suppl 2):S148–58.

24. Borody TJ, Leis S, Pang G, et al. Fecal microbiota transplantation in the treatment of recurrent Clostridium difficile infection. Up to Date. 2016. Available at: http://www.uptodate.com/contents/topic.do?topicKey=GAST/2604. Accessed March 10, 2017.

25. Grigoras CA, Zervou FN, Zacharioudakis IM, et al. Isolation of C. difficile carriers alone and as part of a bundle approach for the prevention of Clostridium difficile infection (CDI): a mathematical model based on clinical study data. PLoS One 2016;11(6):e0156577.

26. Søes L, Brock I, Persson S, et al. Clinical features of Clostridium difficile infection and molecular characterization of the isolated strains in a cohort of Danish hospitalized patients. Eur J Clin Microbiol Infect Dis 2012;31(2):185–92.

27. Petrella L, Sambol S, Gerding D, et al. Decreased cure and increased recurrence rates for clostridium difficile infection caused by the epidemic C. difficile BI strain. Clin Infect Dis 2012;(3):351.

28. Boyle M, Ruth-Sahd L, Zhou Z. Fecal microbiota transplant to treat recurrent Clostridium difficile infections. Crit Care Nurse 2015;35(2):51–64.

29. Blixt T, Gradel K, Homann C, et al. Asymptomatic carriers contribute to nosocomial Clostridium difficile infection: a cohort study of 4508 patients. Gastroenterology 2017;152(5):1031–41.e2. https://doi.org/10.1053/j.gastro.2016.12.035.

30. Delate T, Albrecht G, Won K, et al. Ambulatory-treated Clostridium difficile infection: a comparison of community-acquired vs. nosocomial infection. Epidemiol Infect 2015;143(6):1225–35.

31. Stone N, Sidak-Loftis L, Wagner D, et al. More than 50% of Clostridium difficile isolates from pet dogs in Flagstaff, USA, carry toxigenic genotypes. PLoS One 2016;11(10):e0164504.

32. Johnston BC, Ma SS, Goldenberg JZ, et al. Probiotics for the prevention of Clostridium difficile-associated diarrhea: a systematic review and meta-analysis (Structured abstract). Ann Intern Med 2012;157(12):878–88.

33. Hempel S, Newberry SJ, Maher AR, et al. Probiotics for the prevention and treatment of antibiotic-associated diarrhea: a systematic review and meta-analysis (Structured abstract). JAMA 2012;307:1959–69.

34. Xie C, Li J, Wang K, et al. Probiotics for the prevention of antibiotic-associated diarrhoea in older patients: a systematic review. Travel Med Infect Dis 2015; 13(2):128–34.

35. Szajewska H, Kołodziej M. Systematic review with meta-analysis: Saccharomyces boulardii in the prevention of antibiotic-associated diarrhoea. Aliment Pharmacol Ther 2015;42(7):793–801.

36. Selinger C, Bell A, Cairns A, et al. Probiotic VSL#3 prevents antibiotic-associated diarrhoea in a double-blind, randomized, placebo-controlled clinical trial. J Hosp Infect 2013;84(2):159–65.

37. Lactobacilli and Bifidobacteria in the prevention of antibiotic-associated diarrhoea and Clostridium difficile diarrhoea in older inpatients (PLACIDE): a

randomised, double-blind, placebo-controlled, multicentre trial. Lancet 2013;(9900):1249.

38. Weed H. ACP Journal Club. Review: probiotics prevent C. difficile-associated diarrhea in patients using antibiotics. Ann Intern Med 2013;159(8):JC7.

39. Goldenberg J. Probiotics for the prevention of Clostridium difficile-associated diarrhea in adults and children. Cochrane Database Syst Rev 2013;(5). https://doi.org/10.1002/14651858.CD006095.pub3.

40. Videlock E, Cremonini F. Meta-analysis: probiotics in antibiotic-associated diarrhoea. Aliment Pharmacol Ther 2012;35(12):1355–69.

41. Wright K, Wright H, Murray M. Probiotic treatment for the prevention of antibiotic-associated diarrhoea in geriatric patients: a multicentre randomised controlled pilot study. Australas J Ageing 2015;34(1):38–42.

42. Bernard H, Little J. The impact of ultraviolet (UV) disinfection system coupled with evidence-based interventions on the incidence of hospital onset Clostridium difficile (HO-C-Diff). 42nd Annual Conference Abstracts, APIC 2015, Nashville, TN June 2015. Am J Infect Control 2015;43:S27.

43. Forsman J, Anani N, Eghdam A, et al. Integrated information visualization to support decision making for use of antibiotics in intensive care: design and usability evaluation. Inform Health Soc Care 2013;38(4):330–53.

44. Rodriguez S, Hernandez MB, Tarchii G, et al. Risk of Clostridium difficile infection in hospitalized patients receiving metronidazole for a non-C difficile infection. Clin Gastroenterol Hepatol 2014;12(11):1856–61.

45. Spinler J, Ross C, Savidge T. Probiotics as adjunctive therapy for preventing Clostridium difficile infection - what are we waiting for? Anaerobe 2016;41:51–7.

46. Kali A, Charles M, Srirangaraj S. Cadazolid: a new hope in the treatment of Clostridium difficile infection. Australas Med J 2015;8(8):253–62.

Common Gastrointestinal Complications Associated with Human Immunodeficiency Virus/AIDS: An Overview

Vincent P. Hall, PhD, RN, CNE

KEYWORDS

- HIV/AIDS • Diarrhea • Nausea and vomiting • HIV enteropathy

KEY POINTS

- With the use of highly active antiretroviral therapy, human immunodeficiency virus (HIV)/AIDS has become a manageable chronic illness.
- The gastrointestinal system is a major target of HIV infection.
- Diarrhea and nausea and vomiting (NV) remain a common problem for people living with HIV/AIDS (PLWHA).
- The causes of diarrhea and NV have shifted from primarily infectious to noninfectious causes.
- Diarrhea and NV can have substantial negative health outcomes for PLWHA.

INTRODUCTION

Since the beginning of the human immunodeficiency virus (HIV)/AIDS epidemic, 1,216,917 people in the United States have been diagnosed with AIDS; based on 2013 data, an estimated 1,242,000 adults and adolescents were living with HIV.[1] The development and effective use of highly active antiretroviral therapy (HAART) has transformed the disease into a manageable chronic illness.[2,3] When treated early and aggressively, people living with HIV/AIDS (PLWHA) in the developed world have a life expectancy that approaches those of uninfected individuals.[2–4] Nonetheless, as with other chronic illnesses, PLWHA can experience multiple physical symptoms or problems related to HIV infection and treatment. A common problem for PLWHA continues to be gastrointestinal (GI) conditions.

Disclosure Statement: The author reports no real or perceived vested interests that relate to this article that could be construed as a conflict of interest.
School of Nursing, Walden University, 100 Washington Avenue, South Suite 900, Minneapolis, MN 55401, USA
E-mail address: Vincent.hall@mail.waldenu.edu

Crit Care Nurs Clin N Am 30 (2018) 101–107
https://doi.org/10.1016/j.cnc.2017.10.009
0899-5885/18/© 2017 Elsevier Inc. All rights reserved.

Common GI conditions or symptoms associated with HIV include diarrhea, nausea and vomiting (NV), bloating, abdominal discomfort, and changes in body weight.[5,6] However, 2 of the most commonly reported problems by PLWHA are diarrhea and nausea. Up to 60% of individuals with HIV report diarrhea[5]; evidence suggests that NV remains a significant problem among PLWHA, particularly related to the use of HAART.[7,8] Diarrhea and NV can negatively impact the quality of life, adherence to medication therapy, and eating among PLWHA and are common reasons to change or discontinue HAART regimens.[2,5,7] Because diarrhea and NV can have substantial negative health outcomes for PLWHA, it is important to understand the causes of these conditions.

Diarrhea

Diarrhea in PLWHA can generally be classified as infectious or noninfectious in nature. The origin of infectious diarrhea can occur from a variety of opportunistic pathogens that can be organized into 4 general categories: bacteria, fungi, viruses, and protozoa.[9,10] The occurrence of infectious diarrhea in the United States has declined significantly since the advent of HAART.[2] However, it can still occur in individuals who are significantly immunocompromised and who have CD4+ T-cell counts less than 200 cells per cubic millimeter.[5] **Table 1** provides an overview of common causes of infectious diarrhea in immunocompromised individuals with HIV.

Although the occurrence of infectious diarrhea has declined because of HAART, diarrhea due to noninfectious causes has increased.[2,5] The causes of noninfectious diarrhea include HIV enteropathy, HAART-associated diarrhea, autonomic neuropathy, and chronic pancreatitis.[2,5,10] In order to understand the causes of noninfectious diarrhea in PLWHA it is important examine the pathophysiology of HIV and the GI tract, particularly as it relates to HIV enteropathy.

Pathophysiology

The mucosal surface of the GI tract functions in an anatomic and physiologic role that serves as a barrier against microorganisms.[11] Gut-associated lymphoid tissue (GALT)

Table 1		
Overview of common causes of infectious diarrhea		
Category	**Pathogen**	**Common Signs and Symptoms**
Bacteria	MAC	Diarrhea Fever Weight loss
Fungi	*Histoplasma capsulatum* (histoplasmosis)	Abdominal pain Diarrhea Weight loss Fever
Virus	CMV	Diarrhea Abdominal pain Rectal bleeding Fever Weight loss
Protozoa	*Cryptosporidium parvum*	Severe watery diarrhea Severe dehydration Electrolyte imbalances

Abbreviations: CMV, cytomegalovirus; MAC, *Mycobacterium avium* complex.

Data from Dikman AE, Schonfeld E, Srisarajivakul NC, et al. Human immunodeficiency virus-associated diarrhea: still an issue in the era of antiretroviral therapy. Dig Dis Sci 2015;60:2236–45.

represents the largest collection of lymphoid tissue in the body and is regularly exposed to multiple types of antigens from microbial and dietary sources. Naïve B and T cells in the GALT constantly interact with antigens that cause their maturation into plasma cells and memory T cells.[2] Because of this constant stimulation of the immune system, a baseline inflammatory state exists that prompts the production of chemokines and adhesion molecules, which then mediates the movement of lymphocytes into the mucosal tissues.[12] The GI tract is one of the most heavily targeted areas by the HIV infection and occurs at all stages of the infection but impacts the mucosal immune system, particularly during the acute infection phase.[2,13] Within weeks of HIV infection, most CD4+ lymphocytes are depleted in the GI mucosal lamina.[12] CD4+ cells in the mucosa express CC chemokine receptor type 5 (CCR5), which serves as the primary coreceptor for most infective HIV strains.[14] CCR5 assists the entry of the HIV virus into CD4+ T cells; because they are particularly active in the mucosa, CCR5 supports HIV replication and ultimately CD4+ depletion.[2] Even with HAART, the GALT remains a reservoir for HIV and low levels of viral replication may persist there.[5,10]

Human immunodeficiency virus enteropathy

HIV enteropathy is an idiopathic form of diarrhea that can occur in patients with HIV in the absence of an identified pathogen.[2,5] It can occur at any stage of the disease from the acute phase to advanced AIDS. The pathologic process leading to HIV enteropathy is still not clear, but several mechanisms have been suggested. As noted previously, the GALT is an early and heavily targeted area of HIV replication and CD4+ T-cell depletion. One study has demonstrated that HIV-induced damage to the GALT occurs early during the infection, even before seroconversion can be detected.[15] Rapid destruction of CD4+ T cells also included increased epithelial cell death and the loss of proteins involved in intestinal epithelial barrier and mucosal functions. Histologic changes occur that include villous atrophy and crypt hyperplasia, and inflammatory infiltrates of lymphocytes in the lamina propria can be seen.[5,10] Damage to the mucosal barrier results in diarrhea and can also lead to malabsorption of vitamin B_{12}, bile, and sugars.[2,10,11]

In addition to HIV infection's impact on the GALT, HIV can also infect cells of the GI tract, including enterocytes, lamina propria cells, and the submucosa.[5,11] Infection by HIV of enterocytes may lead to changes in cellular differentiation, villous atrophy, and altered absorptive and secretory function of the GI tract. The toxic effects on cells of the GI tract may also occur because of the viral proteins that are shed from infected cells.[5] HAART generally improves HIV enteropathy, but it is not always effective.[5,11]

Highly active antiretroviral therapy–associated diarrhea

Diarrhea is a common side effect of antiretroviral medications and can be severe enough to require the change or discontinuation of medication.[10] It is difficult to provide a precise estimation of the incidence or prevalence of HAART-associated diarrhea among PLWHA because of the multiple ways diarrhea has been defined in studies.[16] However, it has been estimated that HAART-associated diarrhea may occur in up to 50% of PLWHA depending on their drug regimen.[17] Diarrhea can be linked to several types of medication classes in HAART, including nucleoside reverse-transcriptase inhibitors, non-nucleoside reverse-transcriptase inhibitors, protease inhibitors (PIs), and integrase inhibitors.[5,10] Among antiretroviral therapies (ARTs) PIs, particularly ritonavir, seem to produce the greatest risk of ART-associated diarrhea among PLWHA.[18] Ritonavir is used to boost the therapeutic effect of other PIs and, despite its being used in reduced dosage, can still commonly produce diarrhea depending on the other types of ARTs used in combination therapy.[2,5] Data suggest that HAART-associated diarrhea can be caused by several mechanisms; but in mouse models, PIs have been found to increase water and electrolyte secretion into the intestinal lumen, thus, leading to diarrhea.[19] Among drug combinations, lopinavir-ritonavir and fosamprenavir-ritonavir have tended to present higher rates of drug-related diarrhea, which can be moderate to potentially life threatening, versus other combinations, such as saquinavir-ritonavir or darunavir-ritonavir.[5,16]

Other causes of noninfectious diarrhea

Other possible causes of noninfectious diarrhea can include pancreatitis and autonomic neuropathy. Pancreatitis can be caused by opportunistic infections (OIs), viral hepatitis, HAART, and HIV itself.[10] Pancreatitis in its chronic form may lead to the development of foul-smelling, bulky stools (steatorrhea).[5] Damage to the autonomic nervous system is a complication of HIV infection.[5,10] Structural damage to autonomic nerves in the GI tract have been observed and can occur at all stages of HIV infection, and this damage may increase intestinal transit time and result in the occurrence of diarrhea.[5,10]

Nausea and Vomiting

As with diarrhea, the cause of NV was primarily the effect of some OIs, such as esophageal candidiasis or cryptosporidiosis, before the development of HAART.[8] With the onset of HAART, the causes of NV are multifactorial and can include medication side effects, overlapping drug interactions, and OIs in PLWHA who have poor immune status.[8,20] However, multiple studies have reported that NV is the most frequently reported side effect of HAART and is also the most frequently cited reason for stopping or nonadherence to drug regimens.[7,8]

Pathophysiology of nausea and vomiting

The pathophysiology of NV is well understood. The vomiting center is located in the lateral medullary reticular formation of the central nervous system. This center manages vomiting and can be activated in different ways, including the chemoreceptor trigger zone (CTZ).[20] The CTZ is located in the area postrema on the floor of the fourth ventricle and is directly linked with the vomiting center located in the medulla.[8,20] Afferent nerves in the GI tract sense mechanical and chemical change and relay this information to the CTZ. Because the CTZ is not protected by the blood-brain barrier, it can be activated by emetogenic chemicals, such as toxins or drugs, in the blood, cerebrospinal fluid, stomach, or small intestines.[21] Once the CTZ is activated, a coordinated and complex set of muscular contractions, cardiovascular responses, and reverse peristalsis occur through various efferent branches of cranial nerves that result in vomiting.[20]

Human immunodeficiency virus medications and nausea and vomiting

NV related to ART generally occurs during the first few days of therapy and may ease after the first few days or weeks, along with the lessening of in intensity and frequency of symptoms.[8] However, in some cases, NV can become chronic with symptoms lasting longer than a month and continuing throughout the course of treatment.[8,20] ART drugs may directly irritate the lining of the GI tract, but there is also evidence that NV is a result of the body sensing the drugs as toxins and attempting to remove them.[20] Either cause can initiate the vomiting mechanism noted in the previous section. Despite the cause, nearly all ARTs can cause NV.

The occurrence and severity of NV can vary widely among individuals receiving HAART but can be influenced by the type of medication or combination of medications and the stage of HIV disease.[20]

SUMMARY

This overview focuses on the 2 most commonly reported problems by PLWHAs: diarrhea and NV. The literature on GI complications and reasons for admission to critical care units (CCUs) is limited. However, it has been noted that the most common complication associated with PLWHA's admission to the CCU is a GI bleed.[22] About half of the GI bleeds are found in the upper GI tract.[22] These bleeds are associated with HIV-related conditions, such as Kaposi sarcoma, infectious ulcers, and AIDS-associated lymphoma. About 70% of lower GI bleeding is related to the underlying HIV infection. Management is similar to that of non–HIV-infected patients and includes fluid resuscitation, finding the source of the bleed, and prevention of recurrent bleeding.

Other GI disorders bringing patients to critical care include hepatic encephalopathy, peritonitis from small bowel enteritis, bowel perforations associated with Kaposi sarcoma, lymphoma, and mycobacterial infection.[22] HAART can cause unpredictable GI absorption as well as pancreatitis.[10,22] Careful evaluation in HIV-infected patients with acute abdominal problems is very important.

The use of HAART has transformed HIV/AIDS into a manageable chronic illness. Although OIs historically were often primary causes of diarrhea and NV in PLWHA, the use of HAART has shifted the primary cause of these conditions to those that are drug-induced. Diarrhea and NV can lead to nonadherence, change, or discontinuance of therapy.[16,22] Nonadherence or patient discontinuance of therapy is a significant issue because decreasing levels of adherence or discontinuance of therapy can lead to increased therapy failure rates and increase the risk of viral mutation and development of resistance to antiviral medications or classes of antiretroviral medications.[8] Diarrhea and NV can also have other serious consequences, such as dehydration, electrolyte imbalances, severe weight loss, malnutrition, fatigue, and decreasing levels of physical functioning.[8,16]

After starting ART, the probability of remaining free from adverse side effects seems to decrease over time.[23] As PLWHA life expectancies increase, they may also experience other age-related illnesses that require additional medications; this polypharmacy can increase the risk of medication-related side effects.[8] In addition to the physical impacts, diarrhea and NV can negatively impact quality of life and lead to social isolation and feelings of loss of control and shame.[2,5,16] It has been noted that HIV infection can be considered a disease of the GI tract because it is a significant target of infection[11] and because of the side effects HAART can have on the GI system. Therefore, it is important that clinicians have an understanding of the causes of diarrhea and NV in PLWHA and educate patients about potential side effects and treatment options.

REFERENCES

1. Centers for Disease Control. HIV in the United States: at a glance. 2017. Available at: https://www.cdc.gov/hiv/statistics/overview/ataglance.html. Accessed June 8, 2017.
2. Dikman AE, Schonfeld E, Srisarajivakul NC, et al. Human immunodeficiency virus-associated diarrhea: still an issue in the era of antiretroviral therapy. Dig Dis Sci 2015;60:2236–45.

3. Lorenc A, Robinson N. A review of the use of complementary and alternative medicine and HIV: issues for patient care. AIDS Patient Care STDs 2013;27:503–10.

4. The Collaboration of Observational HIV Epidemiological Research Europe (COHERE) in EuroCoord, Lewden C, Bouteloup V, De Wit S, et al. All-cause mortality in treated HIV-infected adults with CD4 >=500/mm3 compared with the general population: evidence from a large European observational cohort collaboration. Int J Epidemiol 2012;41:433–45.

5. Macarthur RD, Dupont HL. Etiology and pharmacologic management of noninfectious diarrhea in HIV-infected individuals in the highly active antiretroviral therapy era. Clin Infect Dis 2012;55:860–7.

6. Wilson NL, Moneyham LD, Alexandrov AW. A systematic review of probiotics as a potential intervention to restore gut health in HIV infection. J Assoc Nurses AIDS Care 2013;24:98–111.

7. Anderson EH, Delaney C, Hull M. Experience of nausea in persons with HIV/AIDS. J Nurses Staff Development 2010;26:271–8.

8. Anastasi JK, Capili B. Nausea and vomiting in HIV/AIDS. Gastroenterol Nurs 2011;34:15–24.

9. Rossit AR, Goncalves AC, Franco C, et al. Etiological agents of diarrhea in patients infected by the human immunodeficiency virus-1: a review. Rev Inst Med Trop Sao Paulo 2009;51:59–65.

10. Feasey NA, Healey P, Gordon MA. Review article: the aetiology, investigation and management of diarrhoea in the HIV-positive patient. Ailment Pharmacol Ther 2011;34:587–603.

11. Brenchley JM, Douek DC. HIV infection and the gastrointestinal immune system. Mucosal Immunol 2008;1:23–30.

12. Mehandru S. The gastrointestinal tract in HIV-1 infection: questions, answers, and more questions! PRN Noteb 2007. Available at: https://www.prn.org/images/pdfs/267_mehandru_saurabh.pdf. Accessed June 14, 2017.

13. Santos ASAC, Silveira EAD, Falco MO, et al. Effectiveness of nutritional treatment and symbiotic use on gastrointestinal symptoms reduction in HIV-infected patients: randomized clinical trial. Clin Nutr 2017;36:680–5.

14. Anton PA, Elliott J, Poles MA, et al. Enhanced levels of functional HIV-1 co-receptors on human mucosal T cells demonstrated using intestinal biopsy tissue. AIDS 2000;14:1761–5.

15. Sankaran S, George MD, Reay E, et al. Rapid onset of intestinal epithelial barrier dysfunction in primary human immunodeficiency virus infection is driven by an imbalance between immune response and mucosal repair and regeneration. J Virol 2008;82:538–45.

16. MacArthur RD. Management of noninfectious diarrhea associated with HIV and highly active antiretroviral therapy. Am J Manag Care 2013;19(11 suppl):S238–45.

17. Wilcox CM, Wanke CA. Evaluation of the HIV-infected patient with diarrhea. In: UpToDate. 2017. Available at: https://www.uptodate.com/contents/evaluation-of-the-hiv-infected-patient-with-diarrhea. Accessed June 19, 2017.

18. Gupta R, Ordonez RM, Koenig S. Global impact of antiretroviral therapy-associated diarrhea. AIDS Patient Care and STDs 2012;26:711–3.

19. Braga Neto MB, Aguiar CV, Maciel JG, et al. Evaluation of HIV protease and nucleoside reverse transcriptase inhibitors on proliferation, necrosis, apoptosis in intestinal epithelial cells and electrolyte and water transport and epithelial barrier function in mice. BMC Gastroenterol 2010;10:90.

20. Chubineh S, McGowan J. Nausea and vomiting in HIV: a symptom review. Int J STD AIDS 2008;19:723–8.
21. Garrett K, Tsuruta K, Walker S, et al. Managing nausea and vomiting: current strategies. Crit Care Nurse 2003;23:31–50.
22. Crother K, Huang L. Critical care of patients with HIV.HIV InSite 2006; Available at: http://hivinsite.ucsf.edu/InSite?page=kb-03-03-01. Accessed June 26, 2017.
23. Prosperi MC, Fabbiani M, Fanti I, et al. Predictors of first-line antiretroviral therapy discontinuation due to drug-related adverse events in HIV-infected patients: a retrospective cohort study. BMC Infect Dis 2012;12:296.

Gastrointestinal Motility Problems in Critically Ill Patients

Christine Frazer, PhD, CNS, CNE, RN*, Leslie Hussey, PhD, CNE, RN, Mary Bemker, PhD, PsyS, LADC, LPCC, CCFP, CNE, RN

KEYWORDS

- Gastrointestinal motility • Gastroparesis • Ileus • Toxic megacolon • Critical care
- Nursing care

KEY POINTS

- Gastrointestinal motility problems contribute to an increased risk of mortality and impacts the length of hospitalization and medical care costs.
- Various causes impact normal gastrointestinal motility in critically ill patients.
- The high incidence of gastrointestinal complications in critically ill patients requires an awareness of the causation, signs and symptoms, and treatment of various gastrointestinal motility disorders, including gastroparesis, ileus, and toxic megacolon.
- Gastric residual volume is widely used in critical care settings to assess gastric motility.
- Toxic megacolon is a type of acquired megacolon categorized as a medical emergency and includes severe inflammation affecting all layers of the colon wall.

In critically ill patients, gastrointestinal (GI) motility problems are common and can involve the whole GI tract (GIT). GI complications occur in 50% or more of patients in a critical care setting and are prevalent in mechanically ventilated patients.[1,2] Furthermore, GI motility problems in critically ill patients contribute to an increased risk of mortality, duration of hospital stay, and increased medical costs.[1–3] Surgery, electrolyte disturbances, head and spinal injuries, sepsis, shock, burn injury, hyperglycemia, cardiac injury, respiratory failure, hypoxia, immobility, infections, and certain medications (catecholamines, opioids, sedatives) are some of the various factors that precipitate abnormal GI motility.[1,4,5] Some motility disorders in critically ill patients may lead to aspiration of gastric contents and, later, aspiration pneumonia. This review presents 2 GI motility problems, gastroparesis and ileus, which are common in

Disclosure: None.
College of Health Sciences, School of Nursing, Walden University, 100 Washington Avenue South, Suite 900, Minneapolis, MN 55401, USA
* Corresponding author. 7441 Minnow Brook Way, Land O Lakes, FL 34637.
E-mail address: christine.frazer@mail.waldenu.edu

critically ill patients, and discusses toxic megacolon, a severe and potentially life-threatening complication of pseudomembranous colitis.

GASTROPARESIS

Gastroparesis is a disorder characterized by delayed gastric emptying of solids and liquids in the absence of mechanical obstruction.[6] Delayed gastric emptying occurs in 38% to 57% of patients who are critically ill.[1] Although the exact cause of gastroparesis is unknown, disruption of nerve signals to the stomach may be a factor. The commonly reported causes of gastroparesis are diabetes (30%) and postsurgical (19%), but 36% are classified as idiopathic in nature (**Box 1**).[7]

Clinical Manifestations

Gastroparesis presents with a range of signs and symptoms, which include nausea (most predominate symptom), vomiting, pain (burning, shearing, or gnawing), early satiety, postprandial fullness, and abdominal distention or bloating.[1,3,7] The pain associated with gastroparesis is located mainly in the upper abdominal region (epigastric) and is described as constant or nocturnal (occurring at night). Lastly, pain is often reported following a meal (meal induced).[3] In critical care settings, these patients may also be intolerant to enteral feeding.[9]

Diagnosis and Testing

The diagnosis of gastroparesis is based on symptoms and demonstration of gastric emptying delay. The assessment of gastric emptying includes a variety of methods,

---

Box 1
Factors contributing to risk of gastroparesis

- Diabetes
- Surgery
- Head injury
- Sepsis
- Burns
- Shock
- Increased intracranial pressure
- Cardiac injury
- Respiratory failure
- Chronic pancreatitis
- Liver cirrhosis
- Gastric cancer
- Parkinson disease
- Electrolyte disturbances
- Medications
- Obesity

Data from Refs.[1,4,6,8]

and the documentation of delay in gastric emptying is essential for a definitive diagnosis.[10] Scintigraphy, whereby a radioactive substance is administered and 2-dimensional pictures show the radiation emitted, is the most widely used diagnostic technique and considered the gold standard.[1,5,6,10,11] Other methods of diagnosis include ultrasonography, breath analysis, and MRI. In a critical care setting, the most common method used to assess gastric emptying is to measure gastric residual volume (GRV)[1,5] which can be accomplished by attaching a 50-mL syringe to a nasogastric (NG) tube and aspirating residual contents. Another way to measure GRV is to connect a drainage bag to the end of an NG tube and lower the bag below the thorax level for 10 minutes.[4] A delay in gastric emptying is frequently designated when GRV is 250 mL or greater. However, factors such as patient position (low or high elevation of head of bed), feeding port tube location (deeper in stomach body or close to gastroesophageal junction), and inner diameter of feeding tube (narrow vs wide) may impact GRV.[5,10,11]

Treatment

Treatment of gastroparesis includes pharmacologic measures, dietary measures, and restoring fluid and electrolyte balance. Medications impairing gastric motility, such as anticholinergics, calcium channel antagonists, and opiates, should be avoided.[1,3] Medications, as shown in **Table 1**, are recommended to stimulate and improve gastric emptying and to reduce nausea and vomiting. In critical care, metoclopramide in combination with erythromycin is viewed as a first-line option.[1] For treatment of nausea and vomiting, prochlorperazine, a neuroleptic with antiemetic properties, is usually prescribed to patients with gastroparesis for the management of nausea.[12,13]

Gastric enteral feedings are indicated to maintain and restore electrolyte balance and provide nutrition. However, if patients are at high risk for aspiration or cannot tolerate enteral feedings, then postpyloric feedings are recommended.[14]

Nursing Care

Critically ill patients with gastroparesis are at risk for altered nutrition status, dehydration, electrolyte imbalance, dysfunctional GI motility, nausea, and acute pain or discomfort. Nursing care includes monitoring for old, new, or worsening gastroparesis-associated symptoms (ie, nausea, vomiting, pain, abdominal distention, bloating) and complications. Because hyperglycemia impairs gastric contractility, blood sugar levels and symptoms associated with hyperglycemia must be evaluated. Maintaining electrolyte balance is essential, as disturbances worsen gastroparesis in critically ill patients.[1,2]

Table 1 Medications in gastroparesis treatment	
Promotility Agents: Stimulate and Improve Gastric Motility	**Antiemetic Agents: Reduce Nausea and Vomiting**
Metoclopramide	Thiethylperazine
Erythromycin	Cyclizine
Domperidone	Dimenhydrinate
Azithromycin	Prochlorperazine
Bethanechol	
Clarithromycin	
Pyridostigmine	

Data from Refs.[1,3,9–13]

In addition to the monitoring of symptoms, electrolytes, and hyperglycemia, critical care nurses need to evaluate nutritional intake and status because a high percentage of patients in this setting are prone to gastric feeding intolerance (60%).[4,11] Evaluating intolerance can be challenging in critically ill patients because many patients are ventilated, sedated, or exhibit frequent mental status changes, which impair verbalization of GI symptoms.[11] An established protocol for monitoring GRV should be followed, and interprofessional collaboration with a nutritionist and physician is imperative.[4,5,11] Lastly, because impaired GI motility may lead to vomiting or regurgitating gastric contents, measures (**Box 2**) to prevent a potential for aspiration should be instituted.[4,15]

ILEUS

Both postoperative ileus (POI) and paralytic ileus create major problems for patients. Although many instances are noted on surgical units, complications resultant from the development of an ileus can also be seen in the critical care setting. Therefore, it is imperative that critical care nurses be aware of the causation, signs and symptoms, and treatment of ileus.

POI is a frequent complication of abdominal surgery, especially if the intestines are in close proximity to the surgical site or if direct manipulation of the intestines has occurred. An ileus, or temporary stopping of intestinal activity, presents when hypomotility or absence of motility results within the GIT and is not due to mechanical bowel obstruction. The dysmotility causes gas and gastric fluids to develop and increase in the intestinal tract causing pain, nausea, decreased appetite, and abdominal distention.[16,17] Resulting clinical symptoms may range from minimal signs of discomfort to reports of serious and painful incidence.

Although postoperative complications are noted as the greatest cause of an ileus, additional factors can be linked to the development of a POI. Complex dynamics, such as gastroenteritis and electrolyte imbalances, perpetuate the potential for an ileus.[18] Ileus can result from retroperitoneal surgery, surgery outside of the abdomen (extra-abdominal), and as a complication of general anesthesia.[19] Regardless, intermittently decreased propulsion of intestinal content is noted. Rarely does this propulsion lead to an intestinal rupture.[16]

Approximately 5% to 25% of postoperative patients[20] develop a POI, whereas 10% to 15% are noted to develop a prolonged POI following colorectal surgery.[21] Improvement of

---

Box 2
Measures of aspiration prevention

Nursing Care: Prevention of Aspiration

- Keeping head of bed elevated 30° to 45° during feeds
- Assess feeding tube placement at regular intervals
- Assess for gastrointestinal intolerance and report significant changes every 4 hours
- Use sedatives sparingly
- Avoid bolus feed if at high risk
- Maintain endotracheal cuff pressures and clear secretions above cuff before deflated

Data from Kuppinger DD, Rittler P, Wolfgang HH, et al. Use of gastric residual volume to guide enteral nutrition in critically ill patients: a brief systematic review of clinical studies. Nutrition 2013;29(9):1075–9; and AACN. Prevention of aspiration. Crit Care Nurs 2012;32(3):71–3.

outcomes has been correlated with the inclusion of a multifactorial approach to decrease complications that perpetuate longer hospitalizations[22] and hospital resource usage.[19]

Those with a POI usually recover within 1 to 2 days after surgery; the condition may resolve with conservative treatment, such as a nothing-by-mouth status and NG tube suction. An ileus that continues past 3 days is deemed a paralytic ileus.[23] As with a POI, there is no actual obstruction or decreased blood supply to the intestines in paralytic ileus; rather, decreased peristalsis and motility are the main physiologic problems noted. A paralytic ileus can result from trauma,[24] obstruction of the mesentery artery,[25] or toxins that negatively affect the autonomic nervous system.[26] Regardless of causation, ileus has been associated with a higher incidence of complications, readmissions, potential for reoperation, and increased mortality.[27]

Clinical Manifestations

The exact pathogenetic manifestations of ileus are unclear; however, it is thought that the reflexes noted in the bowel wall, specifically those involving prevertebral ganglia and reflexes involving the spinal cord, have the potential to facilitate ileus. Surgical stress promotes endocrine and inflammatory mediators that also exacerbate the surgical condition. Inhibitory transmission responses are noted with excretion of peptides and nitric oxide. These responses serve to inhibit bowel motility through their neurologic impact on the bowel.[23] The signs and symptoms include nausea; delayed or inability for passage of flatus and stool; abdominal distention, spasm, and pain[28,29]; obstipation (severe constipation); and intolerance to oral intake.[30] Patients with a POI are more prone to pulmonary complications[27] and molecular breakdown (protein catabolism).[31]

Treatment

There is a plethora of information related to the reduction of POI and postsurgical recovery. A common preventative measure for the prevention of ileus is based on the theory of sham feeding, which is that chewing stimulates the vagus nerve. This stimulation, in turn, promotes peristalsis and supports secretion of the typical hormones found in the GIT.[32] One type of sham feeding is gum chewing.[33–35] Chewing gum (sugar free) is associated with enhanced motility and decreasing the time of flatus and bowel sounds presentation,[36,37] thus, decreasing the possibility of an ileus. This practice has also been noted to decrease hospital stays.[34] A semiliquid diet added to gum chewing has been correlated with increasing bowel function.[38] Utilization of an NG tube should be avoided if possible.[39] Much variability regarding the frequency and timing of chewing gum has been noted among the research investigating.[34,35] This intervention needs to be implemented after an assessment and prescribed by a health care provider to minimize any potential for side effects (eg, headache, diarrhea).[32]

Pain management is essential with any surgery, and the management choice with abdominal surgery generally includes opioids. Intestinal surgery activates the endogenous opioids and decreases intestinal motility. It is standard practice to include intermittent or continual intravenous (IV) opioid use after surgery to control pain. These opioids typically bind with the mu-receptor in the body and can increase the chances of developing an ileus.[40]

Because of this dynamic, evidence supports using a peripherally acting mu-opioid receptor as the frontline intervention for pain management. Antagonists, such as alvimopan and methylnaltrexone bromide, are suggested to reduce the endogenous opioid secretions in the intestinal system.[41,42] Alvimopan is designated as an intervention to reverse the effects of a POI and support intestinal motility. The side effects from this medication are not significant with short-term use.[40] Alvimopan reduces the endogenous opioids in the intestine, while allowing the exogenous opioids to act therapeutically on the pain.[40–43] Using nonsteroidal antiinflammatory drugs (NSAIDs) can also assist with the reduction of inflammation and management of pain. This effect, in turn, can decrease the need for opioids.

Another measure to prevent or address POI is control of salt and water administered to patients to prevent overload,[44–47] which minimizes the formation of edema and possible organ failure. Excessive fluid intake is associated with a 10% increase in cases for the development of a POI.[48]

Rocking a minimum of 60 minutes per day postoperatively in a rocking chair has been noted as a prevention effort related to POI. This intervention is thought to have a positive impact on the sympathetic nervous system, resulting in the passing of flatus earlier than when rocking was not used (0.07 days earlier than control group with a $P<.001$).[16,48]

Additional approaches to prevent an ileus include minimal invasive (laparoscopic) surgery and early mobilization for bowel recovery. All the interventions support decreased length of stays associated with GI surgeries and complications associated with ileus.[22,45]

Nursing Care

Solid practices of postoperative care are necessary with any surgery. Making sure that organ functioning returns to normal as soon as possible is a key to early recovery and discharge.

Vigilant physical assessment monitoring by the nurse is important when addressing the prevention and treatment of ileus. To do this, a baseline needs to be determined before the surgical event. Dynamics related to the GI system and overall health are important to know so that deviations and physical health resources can be noted. Examples of areas needed to be collected by nurses include elimination patterns and concerns, nutritional assessment, and health status.[49]

Presurgical assessment and comparisons are made to determine the level and kind of changes occurring postoperatively. A history of bowel elimination patterns and any previous GI surgeries, along with any complications, are documented as part of nursing care. Previous complications related to GI motility increase the probability that an ileus might occur.[48] Surgeries, such as lateral lumbar interbody fusion and anterior lumbar interbody fusion, requiring immobilization postoperatively are also associated with the development of an ileus.[50]

Historically, abdominal auscultation for bowel sounds has been the hallmark assessment technique to indicate the return of bowel motility.[16] Although it is still current practice for nurses to assess for pain and tenderness, abdominal distention, appetite, nausea and vomiting, absence or presence of bowel sounds, flatus return, and bowel elimination, these are not key in the assessment of ileus.[26] Evidence suggests that symptom assessment, such as the resolution of abdominal distention, nausea, vomiting, and appetite return, indicates more POI resolution than the return of bowel sounds and passing flatus.[16]

Early and frequent movement and ambulation as tolerated is an essential aspect of nursing care.[30,39,48] Although this may not increase GI motility per se, mobility can minimize postoperative complications. Possible interventions include sitting in a chair, rocking, and walking. The more movement tolerated and the earlier it is initiated, the chances of developing an ileus decrease.

The patients' laboratory findings must be monitored closely to identify electrolyte imbalances. Nutritional supplementation will be based on laboratory results.

This supplementation may include IV support (including monitoring of salt and fluids), oral dietary supplements, and/or foods rich in the needed nutrient. The nurse must anticipate NG intubation for abdominal distention and decompression of gases and fluids,[26] but this practice must be kept to a minimum.[30,39] Removal of the Foley catheter as soon as possible postoperatively supports gastric motility and physical mobility. Nursing care also includes monitoring intake and output to prevent complications from fluid overload[39,48] and to assess organ functioning.

Monitoring for pain and administering opioids is a crucial aspect of nursing care. Studies have demonstrated that the increased use of epidural analgesic and NSAID combinations used for pain management diminishes the need for opiate-based medications that decrease intestinal motility.[51]

TOXIC MEGACOLON

Toxic megacolon (TM) is a type of acquired megacolon categorized as a medical emergency and includes severe inflammation affecting all layers of the colon wall. The colon becomes grossly distended to greater than 6 cm, which could occur in segments of the colon or affect the entire colon (**Fig. 1**).[52,53] TM is distinguished from other types of megacolon, such as Hirschsprung disease or Ogilvie syndrome, because of the underlying causes of systemic toxicity, inflammatory disease, or infection.[54]

Cause and Incidence

TM affects both men and women and can occur at any age.[52,55] TM most commonly occurs as a complication of acute severe colitis, including irritable bowel syndrome, ulcerative colitis, diverticulitis, or obstructive colon cancer. Approximately 10% of patients admitted to the hospital with ulcerative colitis and 1% to 5% of individuals with Crohn disease develop TM.[56] The mortality rates range from 19% to 45% after TM occurs.[57]

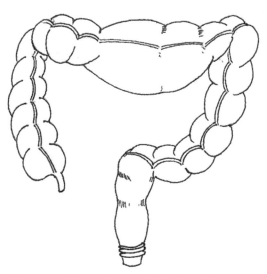

Fig. 1. Megacolon. (*Courtesy of* James Hussey, BS, Naples, FL.)

In recent years, TM has developed from pseudomembranous colitis, which is also called antibiotic-associated colitis or *Clostridium difficile* (C-diff) colitis. Infections from C-diff have become more common because of the overuse of antibiotics and the emergence of hypervirulent strains of the bacteria.[58] TM resulting from C-diff has a 38% to 80% mortality rate.[57,59] Individuals who are immunocompromised are especially susceptible to the development of TM from C-diff and cytomegalovirus.[54,60] Other risk factors for the development and exacerbation of TM when pseudomembranous colitis is present are listed in **Box 3**.

Pathophysiology

TM can occur in those with ulcerative colitis when the inflammation of the colon that may begin only in the surface mucosa of the colon progresses beyond the submucosa into the muscularis and serosa. How TM develops is not totally understood; but the mechanism that initiates damage to the muscles of the colon includes the release of mediators, such as nitric oxide, which impair motility. Nitric oxide is a non-adrenergic, noncholinergic neurotransmitter and is a powerful smooth muscle inhibitor.[61] When the bowel is inflamed because of infection, the macrophages and smooth muscle cells produce nitric oxide. Additionally, the inflammatory process causes the release of neutrophils, lymphocytes, histiocytes, and plasma cells into all levels of the colon muscle layer, which further intensifies the degree of inflammation, dysmotility, distention, and dilation of the colon.[52,57,61] Inflammation continues to worsen as neutrophils cause additional damage in the muscle layer by releasing proteolytic enzymes, cytokines, and leukotriene B[4]. The degree of inflammation and the extent of colonic dilation are related.[62] Microabscesses and necrosis can form. When the inflammation progresses to this point, the smooth muscle of the bowel loses the ability to contract, which causes a section of the colon to become passively dilated.[53]

In an infected colon, C-diff produces toxins A and B, which destroy the epithelial layer of the colon causing cell necrosis and electrophysiologic changes in the colon's mucosa. This effect further increases inflammation.[63] The effect of inflammation of the colon disrupts its absorptive function, so sodium, water, and potassium remain in the lumen of the bowel. Without normal absorption of potassium and sodium, electrolyte imbalances occur, which reduces the colon's ability to contract. The normal epithelial barrier of the colon is compromised, which allows toxins and microbes to enter the bowel and results in systemic toxicity.[57]

Clinical Manifestations

Common signs and symptoms of TM may develop during a severe bout of colitis, which may last for an extended period. Colitis causes diarrhea, which is often bloody,

---

Box 3
Risk factors for toxic megacolon

Chemotherapy

Discontinuation of steroids

Barium enema

Colonoscopy

Drugs that slow GI motility: antidiarrheal agents, narcotics, and anticholinergic drugs

fever, chills, and painful abdominal cramping. The onset of TM is marked by abdominal distention, lessening of diarrhea, constipation, obstipation (severe constipation with intestinal obstruction), diminished bowel sounds, fever, tachycardia, and hypotension.[57,61]

Diagnosis

TM is diagnosed when 3 of the 4 criteria are met based which were established by Jalan and colleagues[64]: (1) temperature greater than 101.5°F (>38.6°C); (2) heart rate greater than 120/min; (3) leukocyte count of 10,500/mm^3 with a left shift, or (4) anemia (hemoglobin or hematocrit of <60% of normal) obtained with a thorough history and physical examination. Diagnostic tests include an abdominal radiography, which reveals colonic distention of greater than 6 cm usually seen in the transverse and ascending colon. Abdominal sonography and a CT scan with contrast may also be useful in determining the cause of TM or detecting the presence of perforation.[58] Blood cultures are needed to determine if septicemia is present. Stool samples are tested for culture and sensitivity and the presence of C-diff toxins A and B. If patients are immunocompromised, such as in human immunodeficiency virus, ova and parasites may be present.[53,62,65]

Metabolic acidosis, volume depletion, and electrolyte imbalances of potassium, calcium chloride, phosphate, and magnesium may be present because of prolonged diarrhea. The erythrocyte sedimentation rate and C-reactive protein are inflammatory markers that can be used to track the progression of the disease.[62]

Treatment

The treatment of TM will depend on its cause. The main goals of therapy are to keep the colon empty, thereby minimizing the stool volume and gas buildup and preventing impaction.[66]

In addition to vigorous resuscitation with fluids, electrolytes, and blood products, medical treatment consists of parenteral corticosteroids, broad-spectrum antibiotics, and close monitoring of patients. Determining if there are life-threatening complications, such as septicemia, hypovolemic shock, dehydration, electrolyte imbalances, and anemia, is a priority of the treatment of megacolon. Dehydration, electrolyte imbalances, and anemia worsen gastric dysmotility, so the need for treatment and aggressive fluid resuscitation is urgent. If patients are in a severe state of shock, colloids are the first choice for fluid resuscitation. Otherwise, IV crystalloids are used for rehydration. Blood products may be required to correct severe anemia.[53,62,66] If patients are on any medications that slow gastric motility, such as antidiarrheal drugs, narcotics, or anticholinergics, they are to be stopped.[59]

Surgery is considered as a treatment option when patients fail to respond to medical management after 48 to 72 hours or when complications, such as perforations or ischemia, occur.[53,67] The type of surgical procedure performed will depend on individual circumstances, but options include subtotal colectomy with ileorectal anastomosis.[67]

Nursing Care

Patients with megacolon need close hemodynamic monitoring of fluid and electrolyte balance, weight, serum albumin, and pain levels. Bowel movements need to be assessed for number and consistency. Stool samples are collected for cultures to identify an underlying infection.[53,68]

Table 2 Toxic megacolon nursing care	
Nursing Intervention	**Rationale**
Reposition to the knee/chest or side for 10–15 min every 2–3 h.	It redistributes air in the colon so patients can pass flatus.
Monitor patient nutrition.	Take nothing by mouth if surgery is needed or if parenteral nutrition may be needed.
Monitor cortisone infusion for patients with IBD and assess fluid and electrolytes (Na, K).	Cortisone medications can cause water and Na retention and K excretion depending on the medication used.
Administer antibiotics for infectious megacolon.	This intervention is for the treatment of C-diff/gram-positive or gram-negative bacteria.
Assess for potential complications 1. Stress ulcers 2. Pressure ulcers	1. The stress of illness causes erosion of the stomach mucosa: administer sucralfate, H_2RAs. 2. Increased abdominal pressure predisposes patients to deep vein thrombosis: administer SQ heparin.

Abbreviations: H_2RAs, H_2 receptor agonists; IBD, inflammatory bowel disease; K, potassium; Na, sodium; SQ, subcutaneous.

Data from Levine CD. Toxic megacolon: diagnosis and treatment challenges. AACN Clin Issues 1999;10(4):492–9; and Mohebbi L, Hesch K. Stress ulcer prophylaxis in the intensive care unit. Proc (Bayl Univ Med Cent) 2009;22(4):373–6.

As soon as dilation of the bowel is identified, bowel rest is necessary. Patients are placed on nothing-by-mouth status, and an NG tube is needed to facilitate bowel decompression. An increase in diarrhea may indicate a positive response to therapy, whereas a reduced number of bowel movements could indicate the bowel is continuing to dilate with an increased ileus.[53] Bowel distention must be assessed at least every 24 hours by physical assessment and abdominal diagnostic tests (radiographs, computed tomography) because the risk of colon perforation drastically increases when the bowel diameter exceeds 9 cm. If perforation occurs, the patients' hemodynamic status will deteriorate signaled by increases in temperature and abdominal tenderness.[53] For more details on nursing care, see **Table 2**.

SUMMARY

Critically ill patients frequently experience complications of the GI system. Complications of gastroparesis, ileus, and TM cause significant suffering and increase length of the hospital stay and health care costs. Moreover, complications of gastroparesis, ileus, and TM significantly influence morbidity and mortality. Critical care nurses must be acutely aware of the high risk of GI complications and provide accurate assessment in monitoring and providing care.

REFERENCES

1. Aderinto-Adike AO, Quigley EM. Gastrointestinal motility problems in critical care: a clinical perspective. J Dig Dis 2014;15(7):335–44.
2. Martin B. Prevention of gastrointestinal complications in the critically ill patient. AACN Adv Crit Care 2007;18(2):158–66.
3. Hasler WL. Gastroparesis: pathogenesis, diagnosis and management. Nat Rev Gastroenterol Hepatol 2011;8(8):438–53.

4. Kuppinger DD, Rittler P, Wolfgang HH, et al. Use of gastric residual volume to guide enteral nutrition in critically ill patients: a brief systematic review of clinical studies. Nutrition 2013;29(9):1075–9.

5. Kar P, Jones KL, Horowitz M, et al. Measurement of gastric emptying in the critically ill. Clin Nutr 2015;34(4):557–64.

6. Stanghellini V, Tack J. Gastroparesis: separate entity of just a part of dyspepsia? AACN Adv Crit Care 2014;63(12):1972–8.

7. Lee A. Gastroparesis: what is the current state-of-the-art for evaluation and medical management? What are the results? J Gastrointest Surg 2013;17(9):1553–6.

8. Nguyen NQ, Ng MP, Chapman M, et al. The impact of admission diagnosis on gastric emptying in critically ill patients. Crit Care 2007;11(1):R16.

9. Gorke C. Gastric emptying in the critically ill patient. Crit Care Resusc 1999;1(1): 39–44.

10. Camilleri M, Parkman HP, Shafi MA, et al. Clinical guideline: management of gastroparesis. Am J Gastroenterol 2013;108(1):18–37.

11. Ukleja A. Altered GI motility in critically ill patients: current understanding of pathophysiology, clinical impact, and diagnostic approach. Nutr Clin Pract 2010; 25(1):16–25.

12. Patrick A, Epstein O. Review article: gastroparesis. Aliment Pharmacol Ther 2008; 27(9):724–40.

13. Hasler WL. Antiemetic treatment for gastroparesis. In: Parkman H, McCallum R, editors. Gastroparesis Clinical Gastroenterology. Humana Press. https://doi.org/ 10.1007/978-1-60761-552-1_23.

14. Van Zanten ARH. Do we need new prokinetics to reduce enteral feeding intolerance during critical illness? Crit Care 2016;20(1):294.

15. AACN. Prevention of aspiration. Crit Care Nurse 2012;32(3):71–3.

16. Massey RL. A randomized trial of rocking-chair motion on the effect of postoperative ileus duration in patients with cancer recovering from abdominal surgery. Appl Nurs Res 2010;23(2):59–64.

17. Katrancha ED, George NM. Postoperative ileus. Medsurg Nurs 2014;23(6): 387–90.

18. Paralytic ileum. MedlinePlus Medical Encyclopedia. 2017. Available at: https:// medlineplus.gov/ency/article/000260.htm. Accessed February 1, 2017.

19. Barletta J, Senagor A. Reducing the burden of postoperative ileus: evaluating and implementing an evidence-based strategy. World J Surg 2014;38(8): 1966–77.

20. Ozdemir A, Altinova S, Koyuncu H, et al. Incidence of postoperative ileus in patients who underwent robot assisted radical prostatectomy. Cent Eur J Urol 2014; 67(1):19–24.

21. Fesharakizadeh M, Teheri D, Dolatkhah S, et al. Postoperative ileus in colorectal surgery: is there any difference between laparoscopic and open surgery? Gastroenterol Rep (Oxf) 2013;1(2):138–43.

22. Nikolian V, Byrn J. Identifying modifiable factors associated with postoperative ileus. J Surg Res 2016;201(2):A9–10.

23. Cagir B. Postoperative ileus. Medscape. 2016. Available at: http://emedicine. medscape.com/2242141-overview#showall. Accessed February 1, 2017.

24. Daniels A, Ritterman S, Lee R. Paralytic ileus in the orthopaedic patient. J Am Acad Orthop Surg 2015;23(6):365–72.

25. So C, Chan K, Au H, et al. Superior mesenteric artery (SMA) syndrome: an unusual case of intestinal obstruction in palliative care. Ann Palliat Med 2017;6(1): 91–3.

26. Nettina SM, editor. Lippincott manual of nursing practice. 10th edition. Philadelphia: Lippincott Williams & Wilkins; 2013.

27. Tevis S, Carchman E, Foley E, et al. Postoperative ileus- more than just prolonged length of stay? J Gastrointest Surg 2015;19(9):1684–90.

28. Vather R, O'Grady G, Bissett I, et al. Postoperative ileus: mechanisms and future directions for research. Clin Exp Pharmacol Physiol 2014;41(5):358–70.

29. Vather R, Trivedi S, Bissett I. Defining postoperative ileus: results of a systematic review and global survey. J Gastrointest Surg 2013;17(5):962–72.

30. Kalff J, Wehner S, Litkouhi B. Postoperative ileus. UpToDate; 2015. Available at: http://www.uptodate.com/contents/postoperative-ileus. Accessed February 1, 2017.

31. Nimmo S. Benefits and outcomes after epidural analgesia. Cont Educ Anaesth Crit Care Pain 2004;4(2):44–7.

32. Fitzgerald JE, Ahmed I. Systematic review and meta-analysis of chewing-gum therapy in the reduction of postoperative paralytic ileus following gastrointestinal surgery. World J Surg 2009;33(12):2557–66.

33. Li S, Liu Y, Peng Q, et al. Chewing gum reduces postoperative ileus following abdominal surgery: a meta-analysis of 17 randomized controlled trials. J Gastroenterol Hepatol 2013;28(7):1122–32.

34. Keenahan M. Does gum chewing prevent postoperative paralytic ileus? Nursing 2014;44(6):1–2.

35. Wronski S. Chew on this: reducing postoperative ileus with chewing gum. Nurs 2014;44(8):19–23.

36. Shum NF, Choi HK, Mak JCK, et al. Randomized clinical trial of chewing gum after laparoscopic colorectal resection. Br J Surg 2016;103:1447–52.

37. Topcu S, Oztekin S. Effects of gum chewing on reducing postoperative ileus and recovery after colorectal surgery: a randomized controlled trial. Complement Ther Clin Pract 2016;23:21–5.

38. Pan Y, Chen L, Zhong X, et al. Gum chewing combined with oral intake of a semi-liquid diet in the postoperative care of patients after gynecologic laparoscopic surgery. J Clin Nurs 2017;26:3156–63. https://doi.org/10.1111/jocn.13664.

39. Lafon C, Lawson L. Postoperative ileus in GI surgical patients: pathogenesis and interventions. Gastrointest Nurs 2012;10(2):45–9.

40. Nair A. Alvimopan for post-operative ileus: what we should know? Acta Anaesthesiol Taiwan 2016;54(3):97–8.

41. Chappell J. Novel recovery pathways to postoperative ileus after bowel resection surgery. Medsurg Matters 2013;22(6):4–6.

42. Viscusi E, Gan T, Leslie J, et al. Peripherally acting mu-opioid receptor antagonists and postoperative ileus: mechanisms of action and clinical accountability. Analgesia 2009;108(6):1811–22.

43. Drake T, Ward A. Pharmacological management to prevent ileus in major abdominal surgery: a systematic review and meta-analysis. J Gastrointest Surg 2016; 20(6):1253–64.

44. Bragg D, El-Sharkawy AM, Psaltis E, et al. Postoperative ileus: recent developments in pathophysiology and management. Clin Nutr 2015;34(3):367–76.

45. Hubner M, Scott M, Champagne B. Postoperative ileus: prevention and treatment. In: Feldman LS, Delaney CP, Ljungqvist L, et al, editors. The SAGES/ERAS society manual of enhanced recovery programs for gastrointestinal surgery. Cham, Switzerland: Springer International; 2015. p. 133–46.

46. Lobo D, Bostock K, Neal K, et al. Effect of salt and water balance on recovery of gastrointestinal function after elective colonic resection: a randomized clinical trial. Lancet 2002;359(9320):1812–8.
47. Luckey A, Livingston E, Tache Y. Mechanism and treatment of postoperative ileus. Arch Surg 2003;138(2):206–14.
48. Thacker J, Montford M, Mythen M, et al. Increased risk of post-operative ileus with excess fluid in the day of colon surgery: results from 524 hospitals in the United States. J Am Coll Surg 2014;219(4):e33.
49. Bisanz A. A characterization of factors determining postoperative ileus after laparoscopic colectomy enables the generation of a novel predictive score. Evid Based Nurs 2014;14(3):69.
50. Al Maaieh M, Du J, Aichmair A, et al. Multivariate analysis on risk factors for postoperative ileus after lateral lumbar interbody fusion. Spine 2014;39(8):688–94.
51. Varadhan K, Lobo D, Ljungqvist O. Enhanced recovery after surgery: the future of improving surgical care. Crit Care Clin 2010;26(3):527–47.
52. Moulin V, Dellon P, Laruent O, et al. Toxic megacolon in patients with severe acute colitis: computed tomographic features. Clin Imaging 2011;35(6):431–6.
53. Levine CD. Toxic megacolon: diagnosis and treatment challenges. AACN Clin Issues 1999;10(4):492–9.
54. Woodhouse E. Toxic megacolon: a review for emergency department clinicians. J Emerg Nurs 2013;42(6):481–6.
55. McMullen TP, Bailey RJ. Advances in the diagnosis and management of toxic megacolon. Can J Gastroenterol 2005;19(3):163–4.
56. Ferri FF. Ferri's clinical advisor. 1st edition. Philadelphia: Elsevier; 2016.
57. Gan SI, Beck PL. A new look at toxic megacolon: an update and review of incidence, etiology, pathogenesis, and management. Am J Gastroenterol 2003; 98(11):2363–71.
58. Leppkes M, Ganslmayer M, Staus BR, et al. Das toxische megakolon. Med Klin Intensivmed Notfmed 2015;110:500–5.
59. Earhart MM. The identification and treatment of toxic megacolon secondary to pseudomembranous colitis. Dimens Crit Care Nurs 2008;27(6):249–54.
60. Beaugerie L, Ngo Y, Goujard F, et al. Etiology and management of toxic megacolon in patients with human immunodeficiency virus infection. Gastroenterology 1994;107(3):858–63.
61. Sheth SG, LaMont JT. Toxic megacolon. Lancet 1998;351(9101):509–13.
62. Autenrieth DM, Baumgart DC. Toxic megacolon. Inflamm Bowel Dis 2012;18(3): 584–91.
63. Halaweish I, Alam HB. Surgical management of severe ulcerative colitis in the intensive care unit. J Intensive Care Med 2015;30(8):451–61.
64. Jalan KN, Sircus W, Card WI, et al. An experience with ulcerative colitis: toxic dilation in 55 cases. Gastroenterology 1969;57(1):68–82.
65. Toxic megacolon. MedlinePlus. 2015. Available at: https://medlineplus.gov/ency/article/000248.htm. Accessed February 16, 2017.
66. Hanauer SB, Wald A. Acute and chronic megacolon. Curr Treat Options Gastroenterol 2007;10(3):237–47.
67. Crib B, Rnajan R, Henderson N. A case of perforated chronic idiopathic megacolon. N Z Med J 2015;128(1422):70–2.
68. Mohebbi L, Hesch K. Stress ulcer prophylaxis in the intensive care unit. Proc (Bayl Univ Med Cent) 2009;22(4):373–6. Available at: www.ncbi.nlm.nih.gov/pmc/articles/PMC2760176/. Accessed February 17, 2017.

Gastroesophageal Reflux in the Intensive Care Unit Patient

Cathy A. Cooper, EdD, MSN, RN, CNE[a],*,
Patti P. Urso, PhD, APRN, ANP-BC, FNP, CNE[b]

KEYWORDS

- Gastroesophageal reflux • Critically ill patients • Microaspiration
- Nursing interventions • Positioning • Acid suppression • Enteral nutrition

KEY POINTS

- The incidence and prevalence of gastroesophageal reflux disease (GERD) is increasing worldwide.
- The number of patients admitted to an intensive care unit with GERD is unknown.
- Current treatment of GERD includes medications, behavioral and life style modifications, and surgical interventions.
- Interventions used in critically ill patients may increase the risk of reflux and complications.

INTRODUCTION

Globally, the prevalence of gastroesophageal reflux disease (GERD) continues to increase at more than 25% in North America and Europe,[1] and notably since 1995, an increased incidence has been noted in Asia as well.[2] The prevalence rate of GERD in developed countries is also linked to age with adults ages 50 to 70 being the most commonly affected. Longer life expectancy combined with an aging population will likely contribute to an increased prevalence of GERD into the future. However, morbidity and the associated economic burden of GERD reaches across the age spectrum, with risk concerns extending even to premature infants, infants and neonates, and those with compromised respiratory health.[3–5] In the United States, the prevalence range for GERD is estimated to be between 10% and 20% of the population, with the most common symptom of GERD, heartburn, estimated to affect 10 million adults in the United States on a daily basis.[6]

Disclosure Statement: The authors have no financial interests, affiliations, or conflicts of interest that relate to the publication of this material.
^a Middle Tennessee State University, School of Nursing, 1301 East Main Street, Murfreesboro, TN 37132, USA; ^b Nursing Education, Walden University, School of Nursing, 100 Washington Avenue South, Suite 900, Minneapolis, MN 55401, USA
* Corresponding author.
E-mail address: cathy.cooper@mtsu.edu

Crit Care Nurs Clin N Am 30 (2018) 123–135
https://doi.org/10.1016/j.cnc.2017.10.011
0899-5885/18/© 2017 Elsevier Inc. All rights reserved.

The specific incidence of GERD in the patient in the intensive care unit (ICU) is unknown; however, it is paramount that critical care nurses possess an understanding of the causes of GERD and the associated risks and added morbidity it poses to the critically ill patient. The purpose of this article is to briefly review the pathophysiology, risk factors, and current treatment modalities used in the management of GERD, and to discuss the assessment of, risks for, and potential complications of undiagnosed, unrecognized, or known GERD in the adult ICU patient.

PATHOPHYSIOLOGY

Specific anatomic structures known as the esophagogastric junction are designed to be protective. The esophagogastric junction is a circular structure composed of strong, smooth muscle fibers of the lower esophageal sphincter (LES) that are surrounded by oblique gastric fibers, which collectively are attached to the striated muscles of the crural diaphragm, and supported by the diaphragmatic hiatus through which the esophagus passes.[1] The esophagogastric junction essentially functions as a 1-way valve to prevent the flow of gastric acid back into the esophagus during varying degrees of pressure changes occurring in the stomach during digestion.[7]

Gastroesophageal reflux (GER), in which gastric contents reenter the esophagus, is a normal physiologic response occurring several times over the course of a day in all individuals. It is important to note that this physiologic reflux occurs transiently and spontaneously in the esophagus for a variety of reasons, most frequently after meals, when swallowing, in gamma-aminobutyric acid–mediated stretch responses, or from gastric distension as a means of expelling gas that has accumulated in the stomach,[8] with gastric distention as the primary reason. GER is also more likely to occur after a large and/or high-fat meal. Intact protective mechanisms involving the esophageal sphincters return any refluxed content to the stomach, and there are typically no symptoms reported or associated with GER.

Reflux that is significant in terms of the amount of gastric contents, that occurs frequently, and that produces symptoms patients describe as problematic or that impact their quality of life, is characterized as GERD.[9] In GERD, regurgitation of the gastric contents into the esophagus is due to a sensorimotor malfunction that results in an ineffective protective antireflux barrier, or additionally, but rarely, from an overproduction of acid by gastric tumors that form in the stomach in Zollinger-Ellison syndrome.[10] A number of factors affect protection of the esophageal mucosal from erosive gastric or duodenal contents. Factors include impaired motility of the esophagus to clear refluxed contents, acid neutralization by saliva, esophageal resistance at the cellular level, impaired barrier function (relaxation) of the LES, and the presence of a sliding hiatal hernia,[1] as well as gastric factors such as delayed gastric emptying (in up to 40% of patients with GERD), pepsin activity, and the presence of *Helicobacter pylori* infection.[9,11] Of interest is that *H pylori* may have a protective role in esophagitis and GERD symptoms, although the association is not well-understood and continues to be investigated.[12–14] Abnormal amounts of reflux can also lead to mucosal changes in the esophagus, including Barrett's esophagus, which is associated with the development of esophageal cancer.[15]

Signs and Symptoms

Efforts in understanding the complex relationship between severity of symptoms and the extent of GERD remains the focus of research. Symptoms of GERD (**Table 1**) may be similar to symptoms of a number of health conditions and diseases. A diagnosis of GERD and its underlying cause may be delayed or even unrecognized because

Table 1	
Symptoms of gastroesophageal reflux disease	
Typical/Specific Symptoms	**Atypical/Nonspecific Symptoms**
• Heartburn	• Noncardiac chest pain
• Acid regurgitation	• Chronic cough
• Hypersalivation	• Hoarseness of voice
	• Throat irritation
	• Globus sensation
	• Increased throat secretions
	• Eructation
	• Slow digestion/early satiety
	• Nausea/vomiting
	• Bloating
	• Epigastric pain
	• Early awakening

Data from Patcharatrakul T, Gonlachanvit S. Gastroesophageal reflux symptoms in typical and atypical GERD: roles of gastroesophageal acid reflux and esophageal motility. J Gastroenterol Hepatol 2014;29:284–90; and Hunt R, Armstrong D, Katelaris P, et al. World Gastroenterology Organisation Global Guidelines: GERD global perspective on gastroesophageal reflux disease. J Clin Gastroenterol 2017;51(6):467–78.

symptoms of GERD may not be perceived as serious or last long enough that an individual decides to see their health care provider or seek care. Typical symptoms of GERD such as heartburn and acid reflux are generally easily recognized; however, atypical symptoms can be overlooked and may result in unexpected respiratory and laryngeal complications in the critically ill patient.[10,16] Esophageal dysmotility has been linked to both typical and atypical symptoms.[16]

Risk Factors

Transient esophageal exposure to acid reflux has been reported to increase with specific foods, obesity, medications, and body positioning. In a large, population-based, prospective study conducted in Norway, an increase in body mass index, smoking, weight gain after smoking cessation, advancing age, female sex, and lower educational attainment were associated with new-onset GERD.[17] A longitudinal study following body mass index in patients over 10 years found that, as body mass index increased, so did symptoms of GERD.[18] Food and drinks that relax the LES and exacerbate GERD symptoms include citrus, chocolate, onions, foods containing mint, and tannin-containing beverages such as coffee, colas, and teas.[19] Alcohol and smoking also strongly contribute to and are associated with worsening GERD symptoms.[20] Medications used in the treatment of asthma such as theophylline, oral beta-2 agonists, and repeated doses of albuterol decrease LES pressure.[21] Nonsteroidal antiinflammatory drugs and aspirin medications used in the treatment of migraine headaches and other conditions, were found to exacerbate esophageal symptoms in migraine headache patients with diagnosed and undiagnosed GERD.[22] Certain cardiac drugs (calcium channel blockers, nitrates) and medications frequently administered to critically ill patients have also been associated with exacerbation of GERD symptoms.[23,24] A list of factors that contribute to GER and GERD are presented in **Table 2**.

As noted, the presence of a sliding hiatal hernia also makes acid reflux more likely. Normally, as the diaphragm contracts, the integrity and strength of the LES increases, especially when bending, coughing, or straining. However, if there is a weakening in

Table 2
Factors that increase risk for/exacerbate gastroesophageal reflux and gastroesophageal reflux disease

Lifestyle, Behavioral, Social Factors	Medications
• Weight gain	• Nonsteroidal antiinflammatory drugs
• High BMI	• Calcium channel blockers
• High dietary fat intake	• Potassium supplements
• Carbonated drinks (especially nighttime symptoms)	• Anticholinergics
	• Tetracycline
• Caffeine (coffee, tea)	• Bisphosphonates
• Chocolate	• Nitrates
• Smoking	• Morphine sulfate
• Peppermint, spearmint	
• Lower education/income	
• Stress	

Abbreviation: BMI, body mass index.

Data from Hunt R, Armstrong D, Katelaris P, et al. World Gastroenterology Organisation Global Guidelines: GERD Global Perspective on Gastroesophageal Reflux Disease. J Clin Gastroenterol 2017;51(6):467–78; and Eusebi LH, Ratnakumaran R, Yuan Y, et al. Global prevalence of, and risk factors for, gastro-oesophageal reflux symptoms: a meta-analysis. Gut 2017. https://doi.org/10.1136/gutjnl-2016-313589.

the diaphragm at the hiatus, the stomach pushes the LES up into the chest cavity away from the hiatus and the support provided by the diaphragm for the sphincter to remain closed, which alters its integrity.

Screening and educating patients regarding risk factors and compliance with treatment are of paramount importance, because untreated symptoms can result in serious complications ranging from bleeding to malignancy.[10] Esophageal stricture as well as nonerosive and erosive esophagitis have been associated with Barrett's esophagus preceding the development of esophageal adenocarcinoma.[10,18,25]

Treatment of Gastroesophageal Reflux and Gastroesophageal Reflux Disease

Because reflux symptoms can range from mild to severe, approaches to treatment vary to accomplish the goal of ameliorating symptoms and healing any erosive lesions. Modifications in diet, such as small frequent meals and avoiding eating before bedtime, and behavioral changes including avoidance of alcohol and smoking in addition to sleep position changes, are part of the primary approach to treatment.[26] Pearson and colleagues[27] conducted a randomized controlled trial testing a sleep positioning device. A reflux probe with wireless monitoring was placed in 20 patients randomly assigned to 4 lying positions after consuming the same meal. Findings were that the right side down position resulted in the most esophageal acid reflux, and use of the device, which maintains elevation of the patient's head, and a left-sided recumbent position decreased GER of acid.

A variety of pharmacologic agents focus on decreasing secretion of stomach acids or neutralizing their effects (**Table 3**). Acid suppressant drugs act to decrease the production (amount) and concentration (strength) of gastric secretions making less available to reflux as well as decreasing acidity of the refluxed secretions.[9] Treatment frequently follows a stepwise approach and is guided by the patient's symptoms. Prescribed and over-the-counter antacids, histamine 2 receptor antagonists (H$_2$RAs), and proton pump inhibitors (PPIs) are most commonly used.[10] There are currently no medications that effectively address the motility abnormalities associated with GERD.

Table 3
Medications used in treatment of GERD

Agents and Actions	Recommendations for Use	Adverse Effects
Antacids (aluminum salts, calcium, sodium, magnesium and aluminum	Short term, intermittent	Diarrhea, constipation
Histamine 2 receptor antagonists Block histamine receptors that secrete acid. Act longer than antacid Cimetidine, famotidine, nizatidine, ranitidine	Short and medium term	Headache, dizziness, constipation, diarrhea Less common: central nervous system reactions and prolonged QT interval in impaired renal function
Proton pump inhibitors Binds to H^+/K^+-ATPase to inhibit acid secretion. Most effective. OTC: omeprazole, lansoprazole, and omeprazole-sodium bicarbonate Prescription: rabeprazole, pantoprazole, esomeprazole, and dexlansoprazole)	Beers criteria: 8 wk in the elderly	Headache, diarrhea, abdominal pain, nausea, flatulence, dizziness and vertigo. Less common: rash, allergic reactions, hypomagnesemia and possible *Clostridium difficile*-associated diarrhea Extended use side effects reported in investigation: osteopenia, acute interstitial nephritis, deficiencies of magnesium, calcium, iron salts and vitamin B_{12}, platelet aggregation inhibitors, increased risk of myocardial infarction, developing dementia Interstitial nephritis
Prokinetic drugs Dopamine receptor antagonist that increases LES pressure to prevent reflux Bethanechol, metoclopramide	Not widely used owing to side effects	Headache, nausea, vomiting, fatigue, somnolence, dizziness, hypertension CNS effects include anxiety, hallucinations, extrapyramidal effects, neuroleptic malignant syndrome, tremor, and tardive dyskinesia

Abbreviations: CNS, central nervous system; LES, lower esophageal sphincter; OTC, over the counter.
Data from Refs.[31,33–36,57]

Prokinetic drugs studied have shown a small effect in reducing symptoms and some, such as metoclopramide, have serious central nervous system effects.[10] Surgery is a treatment option reserved for patients unresponsive or nonadherent to pharmacologic, dietary, or behavioral therapies, or with a large hiatal hernia. Specific procedures include endoscopic fundoplication and bariatric surgery for the morbidly obese patient.[28]

Proton pump inhibitors: Indications and complications
Developed more than 25 years ago, PPIs continue to be the standard of care for treatment of acid-related gastrointestinal disorders, including GERD, and have demonstrated higher efficacy than H_2RAs in multiple trials in reducing gastric acidity.[29] Adverse effects associated with administration of PPIs are few; however, long-term use has been weakly associated with *Clostridium difficile* infection, bone fractures,

and community-acquired pneumonia.[30] Gastric pH can affect the absorption of several drugs, and PPIs influence both absorption and metabolism of some medications. PPI–drug interactions that have been reported include warfarin, diazepam, clopidogrel, levothyroxine, ketoconazole, phenytoin, and methotrexate.[9,31]

Hailed because of safety and tolerance, PPIs have been liberally used even beyond indications approved by the US Food and Drug Administration. However, as more ill effects of long-term use are reported, the 2015 Beers Criteria recommended restricting PPI use to 8 weeks in the elderly, and changing their treatment to H$_2$RAs, because acidity in the stomach is recognized as essential to processing certain nutrients.[32] Magnesium, calcium, iron salts, and vitamin B$_{12}$ deficiencies have been studied in patients with extended PPI use, and complications such as osteopenia, and fractures of the spine and hip have been linked to PPIs,[33,34] as well as diarrhea associated with *C difficile* from altered gut acidity.[35] A nationwide study conducted by Blank and co-workers[36] concluded that acute interstitial nephritis was linked to PPI use. Others presented a case for an increased risk of myocardial infarction, chronic renal injury, infection, and even developing dementia.[31]

Potassium-competitive acid blockers are a newer type of PPI that result in a higher gastric pH effective in controlling both daytime (as do traditional PPIs) and nighttime acid secretion. Vonoprazan fumarate is the first drug in this class, and approved for use in Japan since February 2015.[37] Although not yet available in the United States, a phase III randomized clinical trial is currently in progress.[38] Preapproval clinical studies demonstrated greater gastric acid suppression than lansoprazole for the treatment of acid-related disorders, with mild to moderate adverse drug reactions (mostly constipation or diarrhea) reported.[37]

The Patient in the Intensive Care Unit

Assessment of reflux

There is no definitive single method for detecting the presence of reflux. Traditionally, the most accurate means of detecting pathologic reflux (GERD) is through ambulatory monitoring and measurement of esophageal pH (with or without impedance) in assessing for and during episodes of reflux. Classification of any reflux as acid or nonacid is also recorded. A small catheter is placed via the nares into the distal esophagus, and the pH is continuously monitored for a period of 24 to 48 hours. Patients may also be asked to keep a journal of any symptoms experienced and activities engaged in during testing. The pH of gastric fluids normally ranges from 1.0 to 4.0, with a threshold of less than 4.0 often used to define an episode of reflux.[15,39]

Another diagnostic test is esophageal manometry. Although less routinely done, it measures esophageal and LES pressure, and gastric motility by detecting muscle contractions of the esophagus. It is typically performed together with esophageal pH monitoring, because alone esophageal manometry has not been found to be sensitive or specific enough to confirm a diagnosis of GERD.[28]

In critically ill patients, probes placed in the esophagus have been used to detect reflux as determined by pH; however, because many critically ill patients are receiving stress ulcer prophylaxis with acid-suppressing medications, evaluation of pH may not accurately detect the presence of reflux. Certain medications (such as H$_2$RAs) can result in a gastric pH as high as 6.0. Esophageal pH monitoring is also invasive and may be uncomfortable for patients in the long term.

The presence of pepsin in oral secretions has also been used as a marker for GER. A digestive enzyme, pepsin is activated in the presence of acid from its precursor pepsinogen, secreted from chief cells lining the gastric mucosa.[15] In a controlled, prospective cohort study, Yuksel and colleagues[40] studied use of a noninvasive device to detect the predictive values (positive or negative) for the presence of pepsin in saliva in a sample of 109 patients; 58 with symptoms or a diagnosis of GERD, and 51 with no symptoms served as the control group. In vitro testing using gastric acid samples and sterile water found the device was both sensitive and specific (87%) for the detection of pepsin. Patients with a diagnosis of GERD also had an esophagogastroduodeno-scopy performed and concurrent 48 hour ambulatory pH monitoring after being off acid suppressant therapy for a period of 1 week. Six control subjects and 13 patients with GERD tested positive for salivary pepsin. The authors noted that, for pepsin to be present in saliva, gastric contents must reflux into the oropharynx, which does not typically occur with great frequency in GERD. Another reason posited for the low prevalence of pepsin in the saliva samples may have been that the saliva samples were collected randomly, rather than obtained during an episode of reflux in the GERD sample.

With the goal of making detection of episodes of reflux and prevention of aspiration more comfortable for patients, and easier for the bedside critical care nurse to perform, Schallom and colleagues[41] compared markers for assessment of reflux and aspiration in critically ill mechanically ventilated patients receiving enteral nutrition. The presence of pepsin in oral or tracheal secretions, and pH of oral secretions that contained pepsin were measured in a convenience sample of 15 patients. During data collection, suctioning of the posterior oropharynx (the original location from which oral secretions were to be obtained) caused gagging in the first 2 of 3 patients and resulted in a change in protocol to suctioning only the oral cavity. The authors reported it was likely that episodes of reflux were missed by suctioning only the oral cavity, and there was no correlation between the presence of pepsin in and the pH of oral secretions. Therefore, measurement of pH in oral cavity secretions is not indicated as a marker for gastric reflux at this time.[41]

Respiratory Manifestations of Reflux

Aspiration of small volumes of oropharyngeal secretions or gastric fluid into the lungs without symptoms is termed microaspiration.[42] Aspiration associated with GERD can result from undetected (or silent) events in which small amounts of gastrointestinal fluid refluxes into the tracheobronchial tree and lungs. Reflux aspiration in mechanically ventilated patients is associated with development of ventilator-associated pneumonia.[42] Risk factors for microaspiration are related to the presence of a tracheal tube (ie, an inability of the vocal cords to close, inadequate inflation of the tracheal cuff, and possibly the shape of the cuff), mechanical ventilation (lack of positive end expiratory pressure use and the need for tracheal suctioning), and enteral feedings.[42] A study conducted by Nind and colleagues[43] explored the mechanisms that resulted in GER in 15 critically ill patients on mechanical ventilation. LES pressure, esophageal motility, and pH were monitored 1 hour before and 5 hours during continuous enteral (nasogastric) feedings. Sixty percent of the sample, who were not being treated for reflux, had GER. Forty-six acid reflux events were identified, most attributed to a decreased LES pressure and associated with coughing or straining. From these findings, the authors recommended avoiding interventions or activities that decrease LES pressure, and implementing measures that increase LES pressure may be useful in preventing reflux and microaspiration in ventilated patients.[43]

The association between aspiration, as a result of GER, and asthma was first described in the literature in the late 1970s, with numerous studies to date confirming chronic aspiration of gastrointestinal fluid as a significant factor involved in the exacerbation and development of asthma as a result of altered immune mechanisms.[44] As noted, asthma medications adversely affect function of the LES, and hyperinflation of the lungs associated with obstructive lung diseases such as chronic obstructive pulmonary disease (COPD) and asthma, affect LES function by altering the crural diaphragm.[21] Although there are currently no data to support causality, a high prevalence of GERD in adult patients with COPD and asthma has been reported.[21,39]

A recent study conducted by Tsai and colleagues[45] compared the incidence of admission to the ICU and use of mechanical ventilation among patients with COPD and with and without a diagnosis of GERD. They followed 1210 patients with COPD and GERD and 2420 patients with COPD without GERD for 1 year. The study findings showed that the presence of GERD independently increased the risk of admission to the ICU and requiring mechanical ventilation in patients who subsequently developed GERD versus those who did not develop GERD during the study year.

Nutritional Support and Reflux

Enteral nutrition in critically ill patients is typically provided through gastric or small intestinal tubes. Because these tubes, when placed, impact the integrity of the LES, there is a potential risk for reflux and microaspiration from gastric distention associated with feedings. Reflux and aspiration of small amounts (microaspirations) of gastric contents have been reported to occur frequently in patients receiving enteral nutrition[46]; however, in the absence of visualizing a large amount of gastric secretions in the oral cavity, critical care nurses may not be aware that a patient is experiencing microaspirations. Percutaneous, endoscopically placed gastric (PEG) tubes can prevent reflux associated with a nasogastric tube, and although the LES pressure is maintained (because a PEG tube does not pass through the LES), the potential for reflux is not eliminated with a PEG tube.[7] Rapid bolus feedings via a PEG tube increase both volume and pressure in the stomach, and delays gastric emptying.[15]

Opioids are widely used in critically ill patients in managing pain. Activation of peripheral opioid receptors within the gastrointestinal nervous system results in delayed gastric emptying, and may increase gastric residual volumes in patients receiving enteral nutrition. The opioid antagonist naloxone, administered enterally, selectively blocks the action of opioids at the intestinal receptor sites, without decreasing the central nervous system effects.[47] In a prospective, randomized, double-blind study conducted by Meissner and colleagues,[47] administration of enteral naloxone to 38 critically ill patients who were mechanically ventilated and receiving enteral nutrition significantly decreased the amount of gastric reflux compared with the placebo group.

Stress Ulcer Prophylaxis

The effects of stress on the gastrointestinal system include altered gastrointestinal motility, changes in gastrointestinal secretion, and decreased mucosal blood flow.[48] Critically ill patients being cared for in the ICU are at an increased risk for developing stress-related gastrointestinal disorders including irritation, inflammation, ulceration of the gastrointestinal mucosa, and bleeding.[49] Causes of upper gastrointestinal tract hemorrhage include esophagitis and stress-related mucosal disease. Esophagitis develops from chronic reflux of gastric acid and irritation of the esophageal mucosa. Treatment includes identifying and eliminating the etiology (if possible), and treating previously undiagnosed or inadequately treated GERD with acid suppression therapy.[50] GERD represents one of the most important manifestations of stress exposure to the gastrointestinal tract. It has been shown that stress causes the aggravation of GERD symptoms owing to inhibition of the LES and increased sensitivity to acid, that is, an increased perception of acid reflux. During stress exposure, the amount of reflux does not always increase, but the probability of a feeling of reflux as heartburn increases.[48]

Information from risk assessments performed by critical care nurses on critically ill patients can assist providers in decision making regarding the initiation of stress ulcer prophylaxis. Patients requiring mechanical ventilation, with burns, sepsis, traumatic brain injuries, coagulopathies, or on high-dose steroids, are at high risk for developing stress ulcers; therefore, there is a need to suppress acid production to protect the gastric mucosa. In the ICU setting, PPIs are frequently prescribed for stress ulcer pro- phylaxis to patients. Critically ill patients may also have an increased risk for gastroin- testinal bleeding as a result of comorbid diseases or therapeutic interventions, for example, anticoagulation for the prevention of stroke and the use of nonsteroidal anti- inflammatory drugs in arthritis and migraine headaches.

Research has examined the connection between the brain–gut axis and the effect of stress. The brain–gut axis is a complex, 2-directional communication system involving interactions with the central nervous system (both brain and spinal cord), autonomic nervous system, enteric nervous system, and the hypothalamic–pitui- tary–adrenal axis in helping to ensure and maintain gastrointestinal homeostasis. "Stress ulcer prophylaxis is used in 3 out of 4 critically ill patients."[49(p186)] National and international guidelines recommend stress ulcer prophylaxis as a standard of care in the ICU.[50,51] Summary conclusions regarding appropriate, inappropriate, and uncertain use of PPIs were reported in a recent systematic review completed by Scarpignato and colleagues[9] Short-term (4-12 weeks) treatment with PPIs was found to be appropriate for stress ulcer prophylaxis in high-risk patients, defined as critically ill patients experiencing respiratory failure or with a bleeding disorder. Long-term PPI therapy was determined to be appropriate for GER symptoms that previously responded to the use of PPIs.[9,30] The most current guidelines recommend routine prophylaxis with acid suppressive therapy for high risk-patients, and discon- tinuing stress ulcer prophylaxis if fewer than 2 risk factors are present in the patient, or when discharged from the ICU.[52] In addition, there is some evidence suggesting that a higher gastric pH (>4.0) in patients receiving acid suppressants as prophylactic treatment for stress ulcers may increase the risk of pneumonia and infection with C difficile infection.[53,54]

Effect of Positioning on Reflux

Positioning increases the risk for aspiration from regurgitation of particles of food or fluids in the patient with GERD. The respiratory effects of GER/GERD on mechanical ventilated critically ill patients was previously discussed; however, critically ill patients with undiagnosed or unrecognized GERD who are not mechanically ventilated may also be at an increased risk for reflux when in the supine position, because the positive effect of gravity for returning any refluxed food or fluids to the stomach is absent. Leng and colleagues[55] investigated the effect of body position on GER and intraabdominal pressure in 41 patients admitted to the ICU who were on mechanical ventilation and receiving enteral nutrition. Continuous pH and bladder pressure was monitored in the patients, none of whom had previously diagnosed GERD, with the head of bed at 0°, 20°, 30°, and 45° angles over 6 hours. Reflux fluid type was determined to be nonacid, weak acid, or acid according to pH, and the frequency and location in the esophagus of reflux was also recorded. Findings from the study were that elevating the head of the bed from 0° to 30° reduced both frequency and type of GER fluid. When the head of the bed was elevated to 45°, there was no greater reduction in fre- quency of reflux, but the location of reflux (high esophageal) increased, as did intraab- dominal pressure. The authors concluded that a head of the bed elevation of 30° might be the optimal position for patients on mechanical ventilation receiving enteral nutrition.[55]

Clayton and colleagues[56] explored the effect of nocturnal recumbent (sleeping) position on episodes of reflux in 100 patients with refractory GERD receiving twice daily treatment with a PPI and 100 patients with refractory GERD off therapy for 1 week over a period of 24 hours. Using esophageal ambulatory impedance manometry and pH monitoring, they found that patients on PPI therapy had more episodes of nonacid reflux while in the recumbent position than patients off therapy. Patients off therapy had fewer episodes of reflux, but statistically higher acid reflux episodes. The authors posited that, because PPIs effectively decrease acid production, but do not affect transient lower esophageal relaxations, which can contribute to an increased risk for reflux symptoms, this may explain the higher numbers of reflux episodes in patients while on twice daily PPI therapy.[55]

SUMMARY

Interventions used in supporting critically ill patients such as sedation, presence of an endotracheal tube, mechanical ventilation, enteral feedings, positioning, and medications, along with specific patient characteristics and comorbid conditions contribute to an increased risk for GER in this population. Critical care nurses have an integral role in identifying critically ill patients at risk for GER and patients with known GERD, in preventing complications associated with these conditions.

REFERENCES

1. Herregods T, Bredenoord A, Smout A. Pathophysiology of gastroesophageal reflux disease: new understanding in a new era. J Neurogastroenterol Motil 2015; 27(9):1202–13.
2. Eusebi LH, Zagari RM, Bazzoli F. Changes in gastroesophageal reflux disease epidemiology: a systematic review. Dig Liver Dis 2013;45:S110. Available at: http://www.sciencedirect.com/science/article/pii/S1590865813603059. Accessed May 26, 2017.
3. Jadcherla SR, Slaughter JL, Stenger MR, et al. Practice variance, prevalence, and economic burden of premature infants diagnosed with GERD. Hosp Pediatr 2013;3(4):335–41.
4. Czinn SJ, Blanchard S. Gastroesophageal reflux disease in neonates and infants. Paediatr Drugs 2013;15(1):19–27.
5. Lin YH, Tsai CL, Chien LN, et al. Newly diagnosed gastroesophageal reflux disease increased the risk of acute exacerbation of chronic obstructive pulmonary disease during the first year following diagnosis–a nationwide population-based cohort study. Int J Clin Pract 2015;69(3):350–7.
6. Badillo R, Francis D. Diagnosis and treatment of gastroesophageal reflux disease. World J Gastrointest Pharmacol Ther 2014;5(3):105–12.
7. Lee T-H, Shiun Y-C. Changes in gastroesophageal reflux in patients with nasogastric tube followed by percutaneous endoscopic gastrostomy. J Formos Med Assoc 2011;110(2):115–9.
8. Lee YY, McColl KE. Pathophysiology of gastroesophageal reflux disease. Best Pract Res Clin Gastroenterol 2013;27(3):339–51.
9. Scarpignato C, Gatta L, Zullo A, et al. Effective and safe proton pump inhibitor therapy in acid-related diseases – a position paper addressing benefits and potential harms of acid suppression. BMC Med 2016;14:179. Available at: http://bmcmedicine.biomedcentral.com/articles/10.1186/s12916-016-0718-z. Accessed May 25, 2017.

10. Hunt R, Armstrong D, Katelaris P, et al. World gastroenterology organisation global guidelines: GERD global perspective on gastroesophageal reflux disease. J Clin Gastroenterol 2017;51(6):467–78.

11. Fofaria RK, Morris DL. Hiatus hernia and gastro-oesophageal reflux disease. Medicine 2015;43(4):192–6.

12. Chung SJ, Lim SH, Choi J, et al. Helicobacter pylori serology inversely correlated with the risk and severity of reflux esophagitis in helicobacter pylori endemic area: a matched case-control study of 5,616 health check-up Koreans. J Neurogastroenterol Motil 2011;17(3):267.

13. Rubenstein JH, Inadomi JM, Scheiman J, et al. Association between helicobacter pylori and Barrett's esophagus, erosive esophagitis, and gastroesophageal reflux symptoms. Clin Gastroenterol Hepatol 2014;12(2):239–45.

14. Chandramohan A, Ramadevi AV, Shenoy KT, et al. Association of helicobacter pylori infection with gastroesophageal reflux disease. Arch Med Health Sci 2016; 4(1):22.

15. Ignatavicius DD, Workman ML. Medical-surgical nursing: patient centered collaborative care. 8th edition. St. Louis (MO): Elsevier; 2016.

16. Patcharatrakul T, Gonlachanvit S. Gastroesophageal reflux symptoms in typical and atypical GERD: roles of gastroesophageal acid refluxes and esophageal motility. J Gastroenterol Hepatol 2014;29(2):284–90.

17. Hallan A, Bomme M, Hveem K, et al. Risk factors on the development of new-onset gastroesophageal reflux symptoms. A population-based prospective cohort study: the HUNT study. Am J Gastroenterol 2015;110(3):393–400.

18. Ford AC, Forman D, Bailey AG, et al. The natural history of gastro-oesophageal reflux symptoms in the community and its effects on survival: a longitudinal 10-year follow-up study. Aliment Pharmacol Ther 2013;37(3):323–31.

19. Lewis SL, Bucher L, Heitkemper MM, et al. Medical-surgical nursing: assessment and management of clinical problems. 10th edition. St. Louis (MO): Elsevier-Mosby; 2017.

20. Kiefer DS. Stress-related GERD: strategies for an integrative approach. Altern Complement Ther 2015;21(2):57–60.

21. Harding SM, Allen JE, Blumin JH, et al. Respiratory manifestations of gastroesophageal reflux disease. Ann N Y Acad Sci 2013;1300:43–52.

22. Katic BJ, Golden W, Cady RK, et al. GERD prevalence in migraine patients and the implication for acute migraine treatment. J Headache Pain 2009;10:35–43.

23. Nakaji G, Kogawa Y, Nakamura H, et al. Influence of common cardiac drugs on gastroesophageal reflux disease: multicenter questionnaire survey. J Arrhythm 2011;27(No. Supplement P PJ1_032):218. Available at: https://www.ncbi.nlm.nih.gov/pubmed/21888868. Accessed March 20, 2017.

24. Schallom M, Orr J, Metheny N, et al. Gastroesophageal reflux in critically ill patients. Dimens Crit Care Nurs 2013;32(2):69–77.

25. Ha NH, Hummel R, Watson DI. Endoscopic radiofrequency ablation therapy for the prevention of esophageal cancer in Barrett's esophagus. Gastrointestinal Cancer: Targets and Therapies 2015;(1):111–21. Available at: http://www.ingentaconnect.com/;jsessionid=m0cg1n3lk80z.x-ic-live-02?logoHome=true. Accessed June 21, 2017.

26. Eusebi LH, Ratnakumaran R, Yuan Y, et al. Global prevalence of, and risk factors for, gastro-oesophageal reflux symptoms: a meta-analysis. Gut 2017. https://doi.org/10.1136/gutjnl-2016-313589.

27. Pearson E, Rife C, Freeman J, et al. A novel sleep positioning device reduces gastroesophageal reflux: a randomized controlled trial. J Clin Gastroenterol 2015;49(8):655–9.

28. Katz PO, Gerson LB, Vela MF. Guidelines for the diagnosis and management of gastroesophageal reflux disease. Am J Gastroenterol 2013;108(3):308–28.

29. van Pinxteren B, Sigterman KE, Bonis P, et al. Short-term treatment with proton pump inhibitors, H2-receptor antagonists and prokinetics for gastro-oesophageal reflux disease-like symptoms and endoscopy negative reflux disease. Cochrane Libr 2006. https://doi.org/10.22037/ghfbb.v1i3.33.

30. Yadlapati R, Kahrilas PJ. When is proton pump inhibitor use appropriate? BMC Med 2017;15(36). https://doi.org/10.1186/s12916-017-0804-x.

31. Ueberschaer H, Allescher HD. Proton pump inhibitor-side effects and complications of long-term proton pump inhibitor administration. Z Gastroenterol 2017; 55(1):63.

32. Salbu RL, Feuer JA. Closer look at the 2015 Beers criteria. J Pharm Pract 2016. https://doi.org/10.1177/0897190016663072.

33. Heidelbaugh JJ. Proton pump inhibitors and risk of vitamin and mineral deficiency: evidence and clinical implications. Ther Adv Drug Saf 2013;4(3): 125–33. Available at: http://journals.sagepub.com/. Accessed June 21, 2017.

34. Zojaji H, Bonehy SM. Effect of omeprazole on bone mineral density and frequency of osteopenia and osteoporosis. Gastroenterol Hepatol Bed Bench 2008;1(3):123–6.

35. Tariq R, Singh S, Gupta A, et al. Association of gastric acid suppression with recurrent clostridium difficile infection: a systematic review and meta-analysis. JAMA Intern Med 2017;177(6):784–91.

36. Blank ML, Parkin L, Paul C, et al. A nationwide nested case-control study indicates an increased risk of acute interstitial nephritis with proton pump inhibitor use. Kidney Int 2014;86(4):837–44.

37. Echizen H. The first-in-class potassium-competitive acid blocker, vonoprazan fumarate: pharmacokinetic and pharmacodynamic considerations. Clin Pharmacokinet 2016;55(4):409–18.

38. National Institutes of Health (NIH). 2017. Efficacy and safety of oral once-daily vonoprazan (TAK-438) in participants with erosive esophagitis. Available at: https://clinicaltrials.gov/ct2/show/NCT02388724. Accessed June 29, 2017.

39. Pruitt B. Asthma and gastroesophageal reflux disease. RT: J Resp Care Pract 2016;22–6. http://www.rtmagazine.com/2016/09/asthma-gastroesophageal-reflux-disease/. Accessed March 20, 2017.

40. Yuksel ES, Hong S-KS, Strugala V, et al. Rapid salivary pepsin test: blinded assessment of test performance in gastroesophageal reflux disease. Laryngoscope 2012;122:1312–6.

41. Schallom M, Orr JA, Metheny N, et al. Gastric reflux: association with aspiration and oral secretion pH as marker of reflux. Dimens Crit Care Nurs 2015;34(2): 84–90.

42. Jaillette E, Brunin G, Girault C, et al. Impact of tracheal cuff shape on microaspiration of gastric contents in intubated critically ill patients: study protocol for a randomized controlled study. Trials 2015;16:429.

43. Nind G, Chen WH, Protheroe R, et al. Mechanisms of gastroesophageal reflex in critically ill mechanically ventilated patients. Gastroenterology 2005;128(3): 600–6.

44. Thomas AD, Su K-Y, Chang J-C, et al. Gastroesophagel reflux-associated aspiration alters the immune response in asthma. Surg Endosc 2010;24:1066–74.

45. Tsai C-L, Linn Y-H, Wang M-T, et al. Gastro-oesophageal reflux disease increases the risk of intensive care unit admittance and mechanical ventilation use among patients with chronic obstructive pulmonary disease: a nationwide population-based cohort study. Crit Care 2015;19:110.
46. Metheny NA, Clouse RE, Chang Y-H, et al. Tracheobronchial aspiration of gastric contents in critically-ill tube-fed patients: frequency, outcomes, and risk factors. Crit Care Med 2006;34:1007–15.
47. Meissner W, Dohrn B, Reinhart K. Enteral naloxone reduces gastric tube reflux and frequency of pneumonia in critical care patients during opioid analgesia. Crit Care Med 2003;31(3):776–80.
48. Konturek PC, Brzozowski T, Konturek SJ. Stress and the gut: pathophysiology, clinical consequences, diagnostic approach and treatment options. J Physiol Pharmacol 2011;62(6):591–9. Available at: http://jpp.krakow.pl/journal/archive/12_11/pdf/591_12_11_article.pdf. Accessed June 16, 2017.
49. Krag M, Perner A, Moller MH. Stress ulcer prophylaxis in the intensive care unit. Curr Opin Crit Care 2016;22(2):186–90.
50. Samotowka MA. Gastrointestinal hemorrhage. In: Martin ND, Kaplan LJ, editors. Principles of adult surgical critical care. Cham, Switzerland: Springer International; 2016. p. 169–79.
51. Barletta JF, Bruno JJ, Buckley MS, et al. Stress ulcer prophylaxis. Crit Care Med 2016;44(7):1395–405.
52. American Society of Health-System Pharmacists (ASHP) ASHP therapeutic guidelines on stress ulcer prophylaxis. Am J Health Syst Pharm 1999;56(4):347–79.
53. Marik PE, Vasu T, Hirani A, et al. Stress ulcer prophylaxis in the new millennium: a systematic review and meta-analysis. Crit Care Med 2010;38:2222–8.
54. Kwok CS, Arthur AK, Anibuese CI, et al. Risk of Clostridium difficile infection with acid suppressing drugs and antibiotics: meta-analysis. Am J Gastroenterol 2012;107(7):1011–9.
55. Leng YX, Zhang N, Zhu X, et al. Combined effect of elevated body position on gastroesophageal reflux and intra-abdominal pressure in mechanical ventilated patients. Chinese Critical Care Medicine 2011;23(9):534–8. Available at: https://www.ncbi.nlm.nih.gov/pubmed/21944174. Accessed March 20, 2017.
56. Clayton SB, Rife CC, Singh ER, et al. Twice-daily proton pump inhibitor therapy does not decrease the frequency of reflux episodes during nocturnal recumbency in patients with refractory GERD: analysis of 200 patients using multichannel intraluminal impedance-pH testing. Dis Esophagus 2012;25:682–6.
57. Prescribing Reference Inc. Monthly Prescribing Reference. 2017. Available at: http://www.empr.com/. Accessed June 29, 2017.

Adults with Liver Failure in the Intensive Care Unit

A Transplant Primer for Nurses

Cheryl W. McGinnis, DNP, ARNP-BC, CCTC[a],*,
Stacia M. Hays, DNP, CPNP-PC, CCTC, CNE[b]

KEYWORDS

- Acute liver failure • Liver transplant • Transplant evaluation • Intensive care unit
- Nursing • Transplant complications

KEY POINTS

- Liver transplant has become the standard of care for many patients with acute liver failure or end-stage liver disease.
- Patients with acute or decompensated liver failure require intensive care management.
- Critical care nurses must be able to differentiate normal versus abnormal liver function in order to anticipate necessary treatments.
- Critical care nurses require an understanding of transplant evaluation, listing, and organ allocation.
- Critical care nurses must be able to recognize subtle and acute patient changes indicating early posttransplant complications.

INTRODUCTION

Liver transplant has become the standard of care for the treatment of a variety of liver diseases that in the past would have resulted in an early death. According to the United Network for Organ Sharing (UNOS) there are currently 14,433 candidates waiting for a liver transplant in the United States. In the United States, 7841 liver transplants were performed in 2016.[1] Despite increased education regarding organ donation and advances in patient management, there continues to be a gap in the supply and demand of organs for transplant. Because of this scarce resource, pretransplant and posttransplant patient management remain a key focus in achieving optimal outcomes.

Disclosure: The authors have no commercial or financial conflicts of interest and have received no funding for this article.
[a] School of Nursing, College of Health Sciences, Walden University, 100 Washington Avenue South, Suite 900, Minneapolis, MN 55401, USA; [b] College of Nursing, University of Florida, HPNP Building, 1225 Center Drive, Gainesville, FL 32603, USA
* Corresponding author.
E-mail address: cheryl.mcginnis@mail.waldenu.edu

Crit Care Nurs Clin N Am 30 (2018) 137–148
https://doi.org/10.1016/j.cnc.2017.10.012
0899-5885/18/© 2017 Elsevier Inc. All rights reserved.

Patients requiring a liver transplant often are managed in the outpatient setting but can require intensive care placement for acute liver failure (ALF) or decompensated end-stage liver disease (ESLD). In the intensive care unit (ICU), nurses play a vital role in the stabilization and management of patients before and immediately after transplant. Transplant medicine is a highly complex, specialized field, requiring specific knowledge and management during the pretransplant phase and the early posttransplant period; the best patient outcomes occur when expertise and experience coincide.[2] This article provides critical care nurses with an overview of liver disease and transplant for adult patients with a diagnosis of liver failure.

OVERVIEW OF LIVER FUNCTION

The liver is the largest internal organ in the human body. Weighing an average of 1.4 kg (3 pounds) in average adults, it performs a wide range of functions (**Table 1**). At any time, it holds one-quarter of the body's blood supply, filters 1400 mL of blood per minute, and is responsible for 25% of the cardiac output. The portal vein supplies 75% of the liver's blood flow, and the remaining 25% of blood supply to the liver comes from the hepatic artery. Substances transported to the liver are metabolized, stored, modified, or detoxified and then released into the circulation or intestine to be excreted. The liver plays a vital role in gluconeogenesis and is an important metabolizer of proteins, converting amino acids from foods to produce energy, fats, or carbohydrates. The by-product of this energy conversion is ammonia, which the liver converts to urea, releases into the blood for transport to the kidneys, which excretes it from the body in urine. The liver synthesizes several clotting factors (II, VII, IX, X) as well as factor V and factor XI.[3] It produces approximately 1 L of bile per day.

The liver is the primary site for metabolism of medications through enzymes within the cytochrome P450 pathways. Drugs that affect these pathways are referred to as either inhibitors or inducers; those that cause increased concentrations of other drugs that use this pathway are inhibitors and can lead to subtherapeutic drug levels. In contrast, drugs that cause decreased concentrations are inducers and can cause toxic drug levels to occur.[4]

Table 1 Functions of the liver	
Category	**Function**
Metabolic and nutrition	Gluconeogenesis
	Major role in lipid, protein, amino acid, carbohydrate metabolism
	Produces bile
	Synthesizes albumin
	Activation of vitamin D
	Converts fats to ketones
	Stores fat-soluble vitamins, B_{12}, trace minerals
	Cytochrome P450 pathways
Coagulation	Produces clotting factors II, VII, IX, X
	Factor V, XI
Immunologic	Detoxifies blood
	Filtration and drainage through its lymphatic system
	Converts ammonia to urea
Endocrine	Produces angiotensinogen, secretes somatomedin
	Hemolysis of red blood cells

CAUSES OF LIVER FAILURE

In the adult population, diseases causing liver failure are divided into acute, chronic, or acute-on-chronic causes. In the United States, the most common causes of ALF are viral and drug-induced hepatitis.[5] Acetaminophen overdose causes approximately 46% of ALF, followed by idiosyncratic drug reactions (12%) and fulminant hepatitis B and C viral infections (>7%). Idiosyncratic drug reactions, alcoholic hepatitis, and autoimmune cirrhosis are other common causes that can lead to ALF.[1]

Chronic liver disease refers to liver diseases that last more than 6 months. Chronic causes of ALF are cirrhosis and hepatitis B, because these are the leading risk factors for developing primary liver cancers.[6]

Acute-on-chronic liver disease is characterized by having complications of cirrhosis that has progressed to ALF. A large percentage of cases have unknown causes; however, diseases that cause long-term cirrhosis and often go untreated, including alcoholic hepatitis and hepatitis A, B, C infections, are commonly identified.[6] UNOS has identified 6 categories of diagnoses to that lead to liver failure and the need for liver transplant.[7] **Table 2** identifies these categories in descending order. The trajectory of ESLD begins with inflammation and ends with cirrhosis as the final stage. When inflammation remains untreated, fibrosis leads to irreversible scarring. Ultimately, cirrhosis develops and can lead to a variety of chronic liver complications, such as liver cancer and liver failure.[8]

INDICATIONS FOR LIVER TRANSPLANT

The need for liver transplant is considered when a patient with cirrhosis has signs and symptoms of hepatic decompensation in spite of the use of maximized medical therapies.[5] The most common indicators for transplant are variceal bleeding from the esophagus and/or stomach, significant coagulopathy, hepatic encephalopathy,

Table 2		
United Network for Organ Sharing categories of liver disease		
UNOS Categories	**Diagnosis**	
1. Noncholestatic cirrhosis	Alcoholic Cryptogenic Autoimmune Drug Induced	
2. Malignant neoplasms	Hepatocellular carcinoma Cholangiocarcinoma Hemangiosarcoma	
3. Cholestatic liver disease/cirrhosis	Biliary Ulcerative colitis Crohn disease	
4. Acute hepatic necrosis	Hepatitis B and C, acute or chronic	
5. Metabolic diseases	Alpha-1 antitrypsin deficiency Hemochromatosis, hemosiderosis Tyrosinemia Primary oxalosis	
Other	Cystic fibrosis Budd-Chiari syndrome Total parenteral nutrition–induced liver disease Familial cholestasis Trauma	

spontaneous bacterial peritonitis, and severe and persistent ascites. Once hepatic decompensation develops, patients with cirrhosis can quickly decline because of additional complications such as sepsis, hepatorenal syndrome, and hepatic carcinoma, which are known to increase mortality.[8]

Acute Liver Failure

In the ICU, patients awaiting liver transplant typically have been admitted in ALF or fulminant liver failure, defined as "hepatic encephalopathy within 8 weeks from the appearance of clinical evidence of hepatic failure without a history of previous liver disease."[1,5] Along with hepatic encephalopathy, the clinical presentation typically includes hepatic dysfunction and significant coagulopathy. If left untreated, hepatic encephalopathy may progress to cerebral edema, ultimately leading to multi–organ system failure and death occurring in up to half the cases.[9] Although the cause of ALF can include a variety of factors, the most common cause in the United States is acetaminophen toxicity. Certain anticonvulsants are also well known for causing ALF as well as undiagnosed autoimmune disease and viruses. **Box 1** lists the signs and symptoms of ALF.

CONSIDERATIONS FOR INTENSIVE CARE UNIT NURSES

The role of ICU nurses is challenging, requiring continuous assessment and prompt recognition of unanticipated events. Nurses are critical in providing patient stabilization and supportive care to minimize further complications until organs become available. Key management areas that nurses should consider include ascites and respiratory distress, coagulopathy and acute bleeding, hepatic encephalopathy and cerebral edema, and sepsis.[10]

Ascites and Respiratory Distress

The use of diuretics, sodium, and fluid restrictions limits ascites and can reduce a developed pleural effusion (hepatic hydrothorax). Typically, two-thirds volume replacement is instituted. If ascites is refractory to medications, electrolyte imbalances occur, or dyspnea develops, thoracentesis or transjugular intrahepatic portosystemic shunt (TIPS) may be indicated. TIPS is also useful for portal decompression to reduce the risk of variceal bleeding and is used to improve renal function.[11]

Coagulopathy and Acute Bleeding

Management may require pharmacologic support combined with volume replacement. Daily subcutaneous vitamin K is used to promote synthesis of coagulation

---

Box 1
Signs and symptoms of acute liver failure

- Encephalopathy
- Cerebral edema and/or associated signs of intracranial pressure
- Jaundice
- Ascites
- Hematemesis or melena
- Hypotension
- Hyponatremia

proteins. To reduce portal pressures and minimize bleeding, a vasopressin analogue is indicated. Because fluid intake is restricted, infusions of whole blood and fresh frozen plasma are used. If immediate coagulation is needed, such as in the case of a liver biopsy, platelets may be infused.

Hepatic Encephalopathy/Cerebral Edema

The development of cerebral edema is a major cause of morbidity and mortality in patients with ALF. Increased levels of ammonia greater than 100 µg/dL have been shown to be a risk factor for developing high-grade hepatic encephalopathy; a level of greater than 200 µg/dL predicts intracerebral hemorrhage.[12] The use of lactulose orally or rectally limits the diffusion of ammonia back into the gastrointestinal (GI) system. Oral neomycin is also effective in reducing the risk of worsening hepatic encephalopathy. Renal toxicity and ototoxicity can occur, therefore long-term use is not recommended. Studies that are more recent have shown that branched-chain amino acids have a beneficial effect on hepatic encephalopathy and their use may be increasing in pretransplant patients.[13]

Sepsis

Patients with ALF are at risk of developing sepsis because of the body's limited immune response and hepatocellular dysfunction. Mortality for these patients is as high as 38%.[14] Spontaneous bacterial peritonitis (SBP) is one of the most common infectious complications in patients with ALF. Prophylactic antibiotics are typically initiated in patients with significant ascites or previous episodes of SBP.

LIVER TRANSPLANT EVALUATION IN THE INTENSIVE CARE UNIT SETTING

ICU nurses play an important role in supporting patients and families during the transplant evaluation process. In patients with ALF or ESLD who require admission to the ICU for medical management, intensive, supportive critical care management with liver transplant provides an opportunity for patient survival for most patients.[15] The 1-year survival rate for patients with a primary (first) liver transplant is 91.8%.[1] Patients referred for transplant are seen and evaluated at a transplant center by the transplant team.

At present there are approximately 170 transplant centers in the United States.[1] These centers provide the expertise of a multidisciplinary transplant team approach in the evaluation process. The patients undergo both physical and psychological testing to determine readiness for transplant and the required long-term posttransplant care. The transplant evaluation is a 3-fold process with goals of establishing a diagnosis of ESLD, excluding any absolute or relative contraindications to transplant, and determining the suitability and degree of patient illness to better allocate resources and optimize survival.[16] The evaluation process may vary from center to center with patient-specific diagnostic testing being required; the process may be further modified for patients in the ICU. Common components of the transplant work-up include blood tests, diagnostic imaging and testing, psychological evaluation, and consultation with other specialists depending on the patient's condition. Blood testing includes liver function tests; prothrombin time/International Normalized Ratio (INR); a comprehensive metabolic panel; complete blood count with differential; blood type and screen; viral hepatitis screening; virology screening for cytomegalovirus, herpes simplex virus, Epstein-Barr virus, and human immunodeficiency virus; tumor markers, including alpha-fetoprotein; and arterial blood gases. Patients may require toxicology testing for alcohol and drugs pending the cause of liver disease. Imaging studies include chest radiography, duplex ultrasonography, abdominal computed tomography (CT) scanning, CT scanning of the chest and pelvis, or magnetic resonance angiography if indicated. Pretransplant cirrhotic patients with hepatocellular carcinoma require serial scanning to monitor tumor size and determine treatment modalities before transplant and tumor listing criteria. Additional tests to exclude malignancies may include mammography and PAP testing for women and prostate-specific antigen for men. Evaluation of cardiac and pulmonary functions is also required. Some centers may request upper and lower GI endoscopies to evaluate for esophageal or gastric varices and to exclude malignancies of the GI tract. Consultations and medical clearances are obtained from specialty services such as cardiopulmonary, psychiatry, and social work. If indicated, nephrology, infectious disease, and dental evaluations may be requested before the patient can be listed. Financial clearance is always obtained before transplant listing.

CONTRAINDICATIONS FOR LIVER TRANSPLANT

Contraindications for liver transplant have become fewer over recent years. Transplant centers vary in defining the relative contraindications specific to certain diseases or psychosocial conditions. Many centers mandate abstinence from alcohol, drug, and nicotine use for 6 months before transplant, with center-specific protocols for screening.[5,6] A positive screen can render the patient inactive on the transplant list and may lead to delisting.[5,6] Absolute or relative contraindications to transplant are listed in **Table 3**.

ORGAN ALLOCATION AND LISTING FOR TRANSPLANT

The Organ Procurement and Transplant Network (OPTN) and UNOS are responsible for managing the United States organ allocation.[17] Medical professionals, transplant recipients, and donor families provide input in the national policies governing transplants, following the goals of the OPTN to increase numbers of transplants; provide equity to transplant access; improve waitlists and living donor and transplant recipient outcomes; promote safety for living donors and transplant recipients; and promote efficient management of the OPTN.[1]

Table 3
Contraindications for liver transplant

Absolute Contraindications	Relative Contraindications
Brain death or acute liver failure with intracranial pressure >50 mm Hg or cerebral perfusion pressure <40 mm Hg	Advanced age (center specific)
Active alcohol abuse or drug use	Severe malnutrition
Extrahepatic malignancy	Morbid obesity
Uncontrolled sepsis	Human immunodeficiency virus (center specific)
Certain medical conditions: advanced cardiac or pulmonary disease; acquired immune deficiency syndrome	Multiorgan failure
Anatomic abnormality or thrombosis of the superior mesenteric vein and portal vein that precludes transplant	Cholangiocarcinoma (center specific)
Persistent noncompliance (center specific)	Psychosocial conditions: diagnosis of mental illness, noncompliance, lack of psychosocial support

Model for End-Stage Liver Disease Scoring

Patient disease and illness severity plays a key role in organ allocation and patient listing for transplant. The Model for End-stage Liver Disease (MELD) is used for patients 12 years of age and older. The MELD calculator provides a scoring system to determine how urgently a patient will need a liver transplant within the next 3 months.[1] The MELD calculates patients' scores based on the following laboratory tests: serum creatinine, bilirubin, INR, and serum sodium. A low sodium level is associated with increased mortality, therefore sodium level has recently been added to the MELD calculator.[18] Kidney function is assessed through has asking whether the patient has had dialysis twice within the last week, or 24 hours of continuous veno-venous hemodialysis. The MELD calculation determines organ allocation based on the patient's score and geographic location. Scores range from 6 to 40, with a higher score indicating a sicker patient. Exceptions to this rule are patients who receive MELD exception points based on certain diagnoses, such as hepatocellular carcinoma and portopulmonary hypertension, to account for a higher waitlist mortality not reflected in the MELD score.[19]

In 2013, the Share 35 policy was approved by UNOS mandating regional sharing of livers throughout 11 UNOS regions for patients with a MELD score of 35 or greater. The Share 15 policy provides patients with a MELD score of 15 or greater offers from the local organ procurement organization first and then regionally. Critically ill patients in the ICU setting with a life expectancy of 7 days or less qualify for a status IA on the UNOS list.

Status IA organ offers can be from the local, regional, or national UNOS list. If the patient is too unstable to undergo transplant, the status is changed to a status 7, making the patient inactive on the transplant list until stabilization is achieved and the status updated. Patients listed as status 7 account for approximately 15% of all patients listed for liver transplant.[20] The patient's blood type and size are also required for UNOS listing with organ acceptance dependent on donor-patient size similarity and blood type compatibility.

When a suitable organ is found for the patient, the liver transplant is performed and the patient returns to the ICU for posttransplant management. It is important for ICU nurses to be familiar with potential complications that can occur, often requiring immediate intervention.

EARLY POSTTRANSPLANT COMPLICATIONS

Complications occurring after liver transplant can be categorized into early and late complications. For the purpose of this article, the focus is on the early posttransplant complications. Donor variables known to affect patient outcomes include increased age, long hospitalization, extended warm or cold ischemic times, and donor liver steatosis, leading to reperfusion syndrome, ischemia, and graft dysfunction.[17,21]

Primary Graft Nonfunction

Primary graft nonfunction is complete graft failure immediately posttransplant without a definitive cause.[17] Patients develop coma, coagulopathy, oliguria, hypoglycemia, and marked increase in liver function tests, with transaminase levels often greater than 5000 U/L.[17] It requires immediate relisting for transplant, therefore critical care nurses must be aware of signs and symptoms of liver dysfunction and alert the transplant team immediately.

Early Acute Cellular Rejection

Early acute cellular rejection (ACR) usually occurs within the first 90 days after liver transplant, whereas chronic rejection occurs later. Either can result from low immunosuppression levels, although early ACR is often caused by antibody-mediated factors. ACR is usually reversible but can lead to chronic rejection affecting long-term graft and patient survival. Symptoms of acute rejection include increased liver function tests (serum aminotransferases, alkaline phosphatase, gamma-glutamyl transpeptidase [GGT], and bilirubin levels), fever, abdominal pain, and malaise. The gold standard to diagnose rejection is liver biopsy, percutaneous or transjugular. Treatment of rejection includes high-dose corticosteroids, an increase in immunosuppressant dosing, or adding an additional immunosuppressant. However, patients transplanted for hepatitis C virus (HCV) may be treated without the addition of steroids because of the impact on HCV progression. HCV and rejection have similar histologic markers, often making diagnoses difficult to differentiate. Patients transplanted with a diagnosis of autoimmune hepatitis may require a more aggressive approach to the treatment of rejection, including high-dose steroids. It is important to differentiate rejection from infection in the patients early after liver transplant to ensure appropriate treatment.

Vascular Complications

Hepatic artery thrombosis

Hepatic artery thrombosis has been estimated to occur in 4% to 12% of adult liver transplants and is associated with high morbidity and mortality.[17] Typical causes include hepatic artery narrowing, kinking, and a mismatch with the donor-recipient vessels.[22] Hepatic artery thrombosis presents with sudden and sharp increase in alanine transaminase (ALT)/aspartate transaminase (AST), often greater than 5000 U/L. Bilirubin levels also have a rapid increase, but then quickly trend down because of the death of the hepatic cells. Hepatic artery thrombosis is diagnosed through Doppler ultrasonography. Retransplant is indicated if blood flow cannot be restored to the transplanted graft.

Portal vein thrombosis

Portal vein thrombosis (PVT) occurs in approximately 1% to 13% of liver transplant recipients and can be the result of technical problems during the time of surgery, thrombus formation, or a hypercoagulable state.[22] A PVT can be diagnosed through ultrasonography showing an increase in velocity within the portal vein, CT scanning, or magnetic resonance venography. Treatment may include a thrombectomy, TIPS, or retransplant.

Biliary Complications

Approximately 13% to 19% of adults receiving a deceased donor liver transplant can have biliary complications, which are a source of morbidity after liver transplant.[21] Biliary complications include leaks, strictures, and bilomas. Liver transplant requires biliary reconstruction, connecting the donor common hepatic duct to the recipient bile duct (end-to-end choledochostomy) or connecting the donor common bile duct to a portion of the recipient's jejunum (Roux-en-Y choledochojejunostomy). The type of biliary reconstruction is determined by surgeon preference, underlying liver disease, donor and recipient bile duct size, or previous surgeries.[23] Use of a temporary biliary stent for an end-to-end biliary connection is also determined by transplant surgeon preference. Depending on stent placement technique, the stent may be passed through the GI track or require removal through an endoscopic retrograde cholangiopancreatography (ERCP) around 3 months posttransplant. The stent is radiopaque with placement or migration confirmed on abdominal radiograph.

Biliary leaks and strictures

ICU nurses are more concerned about biliary leaks in the immediate postoperative period. Early biliary leaks are usually a result of technical issues, including lack of perfusion from the hepatic artery, occur at the biliary anastomosis, and the incidence has been reported to be as high as 30%.[17] The patient may develop fever, abdominal pain, and increase in transaminase levels, including bilirubin and GGT. AST and ALT levels are increased; proportionally higher increase in AST is seen.[24] Prothrombin time is also increased. Imaging with ultrasonography, cholangiogram, or magnetic resonance cholangiopancreatography, may show peritonitis or fluid collections. ERCP is performed for patients with a choledochocholedochostomy and requiring biliary stent placement. Depending on the type of stent (plastic or metal), the stent is removed or exchanged within 3 to 6 months. Biliary strictures can be at the site of the anastomosis, usually occurring within the first 6 to 12 months posttransplant.

Bilomas

A biloma can occur from biliary necrosis caused by hepatic artery thrombosis. Bilomas can be perihepatic or within the hepatic parenchyma. Treatment may include antibiotics, percutaneous drainage, or surgical repair.

Infection

During the early posttransplant period, patients are at greatest risk for infections because of high levels of immunosuppression. Most deaths caused by infection occur within the first 3 months after the transplant event, with the highest rate occurring within 30 days.[9,25] Prompt and aggressive evaluation of fevers with rapid initiation of treatment is indicated.[17] Opportunistic and nosocomial infections are prevalent. Nosocomial infections result from central vascular access, indwelling catheters and drainage tubes, surgical complications, wound infections, and prolonged mechanical ventilation. *Clostridium difficile* infection is common because of immunosuppression and antibiotic treatments. Although donors are screened for infections before transplant, consider the possibility of a donor infection if the patient has unexplained symptoms. Infection prophylaxis is started during hospitalization, with length of treatment per transplant center protocols (**Table 4**).

Renal Dysfunction

Hypovolemia during the transplant event coupled with high levels of immunosuppressant agents with known renal toxicity can cause worsening of kidney function. Calcineurin inhibitors have known nephrotoxic effects and immunosuppression needs to be modified in the setting of worsening kidney function. It is important for ICU nurses to monitor for signs and symptoms of renal dysfunction. In some instances, short-term dialysis is necessary.

Table 4
Early posttransplant prophylaxis

Infection	Prophylaxis
Pneumocystis jiroveci (formerly *Pneumocystis carinii*) pneumonia	Trimethoprim-sulfamethoxazole 6–12 mo If allergic use pentamidine, dapsone
Cytomegalovirus	Ganciclovir (intravenous) or valganciclovir (oral)
Candida	Antifungal, such as fluconazole, Mycelex, nystatin

Table 5 Immunosuppressive agents	
Drug	**Class**
Cyclosporine	Calcineurin inhibitor
Tacrolimus	Calcineurin inhibitor
Sirolimus or everolimus	Inhibitor of mechanistic target of rapamycin
Mycophenolate mofetil	Inhibitor of mechanistic target of rapamycin
Azathioprine	Inhibitor of mechanistic target of rapamycin
Prednisone	Corticosteroid

ADDITIONAL COMPLICATIONS

Postoperative nursing management includes patient assessment for bleeding, wound infection or dehiscence, and neurologic changes. Coagulopathy and encephalopathy should improve as liver function normalizes. Careful monitoring of the patient's mental status is required with subtle changes noted. High immunosuppression levels or electrolyte imbalances can cause seizure activity.

IMMUNOSUPPRESSION

Common immunosuppressant agents are listed in **Table 5**. Transplant centers have specific protocols for immunosuppression dosing, monitoring, and therapeutic drug levels related to posttransplant time periods.

LONG-TERM FOLLOW-UP

Long-term management of liver transplant patients is a joint venture between the patient's primary care provider in the local community and the transplant center. Comanagement can ensure the best patient outcomes. Transplant centers have specific protocols for the timing of transplant laboratory tests, including immunosuppression levels, protocol liver biopsies, and specific diagnostic testing based on the patient's diagnosis at time of transplant. Primary care providers are involved with providing preventive care and managing complications of long-term immunosuppression. Transplant patients must be monitored and treated for renal insufficiency, hypertension, hyperglycemia, malignancies, and disease recurrence (HCV/HBV).

SUMMARY

Management of patients with liver disorders in the ICU is challenging. It requires enhanced critical support using a multidisciplinary team approach. Strict monitoring and assessment of the patient's status of vital signs, laboratory values, signs and symptom of organ dysfunction, and neurologic function is imperative to reduce the impact of adverse events before and after liver transplant. ICU nurses play a key role in improving graft survival and patient outcomes through rapid recognition and intervention of complications.

REFERENCES

1. United Network for Organ Sharing [US]. Available at: https://www.unos.org/data/. Accessed June 11, 2017.

2. Gaglio PJ, Brown RS. Who should treat liver transplant patients: the transplant hepatologist or the gastroenterologist? J Hepatol 2006;44:655–7.
3. Northup PG, Caldwell SH. Coagulation in liver disease: a guide for the clinician. Clin Gastroenterol Hepatol 2013;11:1064–74.
4. McDonnell AM, Dang CH. Basic review of the cytochrome P450 system. J Adv Pract Oncol 2013;4:263–8.
5. Martin P, DiMartini A, Feng S, et al. Evaluation for liver transplantation in adults: 2013 practice guideline by the American Association for the Study of Liver Diseases and the American Society of Transplantation. Hepatology 2014;59:1144–65.
6. American Liver Foundation. The progression of liver disease. 2016. Available at: http://www.liverfoundation.org/abouttheliver/info/progression/. Accessed December 6, 2016.
7. US Department of Health and Human Services. National data. In: Organ Procurement and Transplantation Network. 2017. Available at: https://optn.transplant.hrsa.gov/data/view-data-reports/national-data/. Accessed June 21, 2017.
8. Gossens N, Nakagawa S, Hoshida Y. Molecular prognostic predication in liver cirrhosis. World J Gastroenterol 2015;21:10262–73.
9. Bernal MD, Wendon MB. Acute liver failure. N Engl J Med 2013;369:2525–34.
10. Patton H, Misel M, Gish R. Acute liver failure in adults: an evidence-based management protocol for clinicians. Gastroenterol Hepatol 2012;8:161–212.
11. Vilstrup H, Amodio P, Bajaj J, et al. Hepatic encephalopathy in chronic liver disease: 2014 practice guideline. 2014. Available at: https://www.aasld.org/sites/default/files/guideline_documents/hepaticencephenhanced.pdf. Accessed June 15, 2017.
12. Gluud L, Dam G, Les I, et al. Branched-chain amino acids for people with hepatic encephalopathy. In: The Cochrane Library. 2017. Available at: http://www.cochrane.org/CD001939/LIVER_branched-chain-amino-acids-improve-symptoms-hepatic-encephalopathy. Accessed June 7, 2017.
13. Sundeep JP, Amarapurkar DN. Role of TIPS in improving survival of patients with decompensated liver disease. Int J Hepatol 2011. https://doi.org/10.4061/2011/398291.
14. Arvaniti V, D'Amico G, Fede G, et al. Infections in patients with cirrhosis increase mortality four-fold and should be used in determining prognosis. Gastroenterology 2010;139:1246–56.
15. Nyckowski P, Skwarek S, Zieniewicz K, et al. Orthotopic liver transplantation for fulminant hepatic failure. Transplant Proc 2006;38:219–20.
16. Arvelakis A, Katz J, Manzarbeitia C. Liver transplantation workup. In: Medscape clinical procedures. 2015. Available at: http://emedicine.medscape.com/article/431783-workup. Accessed June 15, 2017.
17. Rudow D, Goldstein M. Critical care management of the liver transplant recipient. Crit Care Nurs Q 2008;31(3):232–43.
18. Martin EF, O'Brien C. Update on MELD and organ allocation. Clin Liver Dis 2014;5(4):105–7.
19. United Network for Organ Sharing. Board approves national liver review board and patient guidance. In: Newsroom. 2017. Available at: https://www.transplantpro.org/news/board-approves-national-liver-review-board-and-patient-guidance/. Accessed June 1, 2017.
20. Hansen L, Yan Y, Rosenkranz S. The power of the liver transplantation waiting list: a case presentation. Am J Crit Care 2014;23(6):510–5.

21. Wertheim JA, Petrowsky H, Saab S, et al. Major challenges limiting liver transplantation in the United States. Am J Transplant 2011;11(9):1773–84.

22. Russ P, Garg K. Imaging of liver transplant complications. In: Medscape radiology. 2015. Available at: http://emedicine.medscape.com/article/375855-overview#a2. Accessed June 19, 2017.

23. Kochhar G, Parungao JM, Hanouneh IA, et al. Biliary complications following liver transplantation. World J Gastroenterol 2013;19(19):2841–6.

24. Bonheur JL, Ells PF. Biliary obstruction workup. In: Medscape gastroenterology. 2016. Available at: http://emedicine.medscape.com/article/187001-workup. Accessed June 21, 2017.

25. Kim SI. Bacterial infection after liver transplantation. World J Gastroenterol 2014; 28:6211–20.

Escherichia coli Complications in Pediatric Critical Care

Suzanne S. Puentes, BSN, RN, CCRN,[a],*,
Michele Dunstan, MSN, RN, CCRN,[b]

KEYWORDS

- Shiga toxin–producing *E coli* (STEC) • Enterohemorrhagic *E coli* (EHEC)
- Hemolytic uremic syndrome • HUS • *Escherichia coli* • *E coli* • Diarrhea • Children

KEY POINTS

- *Escherichia coli* is a bacterium commonly found in the intestines of animals and people and is an important part of the intestinal tract, but has the potential to be pathogenic.
- Pathogenic diarrhea causing *E coli* are commonly transmitted through contact with animals, persons, or contaminated water or food.
- Young children are at highest risk and are prone to develop a complication of Shiga toxin–producing *E coli*, hemolytic uremic syndrome (HUS).
- HUS is a clinical syndrome characterized by macroangiopathic hemolytic anemia, thrombocytopenia, and acute renal failure.
- Care of patients with HUS is supportive and requires early diagnosis and treatment in the acute phase of the syndrome.

INTRODUCTION

Escherichia coli is a common bacterium found in the intestines of animals and people. In most cases, it is a part of the healthy human intestines; however, there are pathogenic *E coli* that can cause diarrhea and other systemic illnesses. The most common pathogenic *E coli* are the Shiga toxin–producing *E coli* (STEC), also known as enterohemorrhagic *E coli* (EHEC). Of the STEC, 0157 is the strain that is most commonly associated with outbreaks of *E coli* illness in North America, being responsible for about 95,400 STEC infections each year in the United States alone.[1]

Disclosure: The authors have no financial interests, affiliations, or conflicts of interest that relate to the publication of this material.
[a] Children's Emergency Room, Lehigh Valley Health Network, 1210 South Cedar Crest Boulevard, Allentown, PA 18103, USA; [b] Lehigh Valley Health Network, 1210 South Cedar Crest Boulevard, Allentown, PA 18103, USA
* Corresponding author.
E-mail address: Suzanne_S.Puentes@lvhn.org

Crit Care Nurs Clin N Am 30 (2018) 149–156
https://doi.org/10.1016/j.cnc.2017.10.013
0899-5885/18/© 2017 Elsevier Inc. All rights reserved.

ccnursing.theclinics.com

Transmission of STEC occurs through ingestion of contaminated water or food, or through contact with infected animals or people. The organism has the ability to survive in a low-pH environment, can grow in a variety of foods, and requires only a low dose for infection. Common contaminated foods associated with STEC outbreaks include undercooked beef, leafy greens and other raw produce, soybeans, and unpasteurized juice or cider.[2]

Secondary transmission through human spread has been documented in day care and chronic care facilities. Once ingested, the Shiga toxin has the ability to attach to and efface human enterocytes, resulting in endothelial damage, causing bloody diarrhea. The Shiga toxin then has the ability to disseminate into the bloodstream. Although it does not typically cause bacteremia, once disseminated into the blood stream, the toxin can cause damage to other organs, specifically the kidneys. The renal endothelial cells are injured, which activates the coagulation centers, resulting in the potentially life-threatening illness, hemolytic uremic syndrome (HUS).

HUS is a clinical syndrome characterized by macroangiopathic hemolytic anemia, thrombocytopenia, and acute renal failure.[2] Although acute renal failure in children is rare, HUS is the most common cause. Incidence rate is 0.78 per 100,000 population in children less than 18 years of age and 2.01 per 100,000 in children less than 5 years of age.[3] At present, there is no treatment option available to inactivate the toxin once ingested, or to stop the progression of events once the toxin binds to the receptors. For this reason, the care of patients with HUS is supportive and requires early diagnosis and treatment in the acute phase of the syndrome.

DISCUSSION
Diagnosis

Early diagnosis and treatment are essential to identify potential complications from EHEC, such as dehydration and the more life-threatening illness, HUS. A thorough history and physical is important for diagnosis. Presentation of infection with EHEC typically presents 3 days after ingestion of the toxin but can range from 2 to 12 days.[4] Patients typically present with abdominal pain, cramping, nausea, and watery diarrhea. In many cases, the watery diarrhea progresses to bloody diarrhea. Patients may or may not present with fever and often, because of the diarrhea, patients have signs of dehydration. Social history is important and helps to identify possible exposure to EHEC. Primary mode of transmission of the EHEC infection is through ingestion of contaminated food or water, the most common food sources being undercooked ground beef, raw produce, dairy products, or unpasteurized juice and cider. Secondary modes of transmission that have been reported include person-to-person transmission, most commonly in homes shared with the infected persons, child care settings, or institutional settings. History should also include exposure to farm settings, where cattle, sheep, and goats can be carriers.

Differential diagnosis when evaluating patients with the symptoms described earlier include infection with other intestinal pathogens, such as *Salmonella* or *Shigella*; intussusception; inflammatory bowel disease; mesenteric ischemia; and other sources of acute diarrhea in children. A stool sample should be taken and a culture should be done specifically for 0157 STEC. Patients with high suspicion for EHEC should be placed in isolation until a final diagnosis is made. An earlier confirmed diagnosis allows for reporting to the local public health department. The public health department plays an essential role in identifying the sources, monitoring the exposure, and reporting public information with regard to the contaminated source. Timely reporting helps to make the public aware of a contamination and helps to reduce the extent of the outbreak. One of the most recent multistate outbreaks specific to *E coli* 0157:H7 occurred from January to April 2017.[5] The investigation determined the sources to be a SoyNut Butter product and the exposure crossed 12 states.[5] A total of 32 people were infected, with 12 people being hospitalized.[5] Of the 12 hospitalized, 9 developed HUS, and no deaths were reported.[5] Most of the people affected (81%) were less than 18 years of age.[5] Although the outbreak investigation is over, there may be people unaware of the contaminated product and so there is a possibility of exposure, reinforcing the importance of notifying the public health department as soon as an EHEC infection is confirmed.[5]

With EHEC infection, the symptoms are often self-limiting and resolve with supportive care, but 10% to 15% of patients have the complication of HUS.[1] Again, an early diagnosis of EHEC helps to identify factors that place the patient at risk for developing HUS. Risk factors for developing HUS include age less than 10 years; increased white blood cell count; use of antimotility agents; and increased levels of thrombin fragments, D-dimer, and plasminogen activator inhibitor on presentation.[3]

Although EHEC infection often has providers considering antibiotic treatment, antibiotic therapy for the treatment of STEC is controversial and may increase risk of HUS. A multistate, multicenter, multiyear prospective study showed that, after the first 7 days of the onset of diarrhea caused by *E coli* O157:H7, the development of HUS occurred in patients who were treated with antibiotics.[6] An explanation of this phenomenon is that the antibiotic-induced injury to the bacterial membrane may cause a large release of the preformed toxin.[7] Although there is no strong evidence, a meta-analysis of the research by Freedman and colleagues[8] concluded that, with elimination of bias in the studies and an acceptable definition of HUS, there is a significant association of increased risk, and they do not recommend the use of antibiotics.

HEMOLYTIC UREMIC SYNDROME

The clinical course of HUS is variable from subclinical to life threatening. HUS is a systemic complication that results from the circulating Shiga toxin. Although the toxin is carried through the bloodstream to various organs, including the kidneys, it is rarely associated with bacteremia. Simplified, the toxin binds to receptors, resulting in endothelial cell death, resulting in a triad of macroangiopathic hemolytic anemia, thrombocytopenia, and acute renal failure. Presenting symptoms are a result of this cascade of events. Symptoms of HUS typically present 7 to 10 days after exposure to the Shiga toxin. Since HUS was diagnosed in 1982, mortality has decreased because of early recognition and supportive treatment.[3] Therefore, it is important that, while waiting for a confirmed culture of a Shiga toxin EHEC, patients are monitored for symptoms of HUS and that supportive treatment is implemented early.

Early symptoms of HUS (**Table 1**) include bloody diarrhea, lethargy, fever, vomiting, abdominal tenderness, and dehydration. Late symptoms with which patients may present are a result of the triad of events of hemolytic anemia, thrombocytopenia, and renal failure. The symptoms to watch for include pallor; petechiae; bruising; swelling of the hands, face, or extremities; oligoanuria; jaundice; and change in mental status.[3,9]

Criteria for diagnosis of HUS include hemolytic anemia with a hematocrit less than 30% with evidence of erythrocyte destruction on peripheral blood smear, platelet count less than 150×10^9/L, and serum creatinine level greater than the upper limit for age.[3] Sepsis needs to be ruled out as a source for coagulopathy, therefore blood cultures are recommended. Abnormalities in blood work often include decreased

Table 1
Signs and symptoms of hemolytic uremic syndrome

Early Signs/Symptoms	Later Signs/Symptoms	Laboratory Values
Bloody diarrhea	Pallor	Increased BUN/creatinine levels
Fever	Bruising	Decreased platelet count
Lethargy	Swelling of hands, feet, face	Blood and protein in urine
Vomiting	Oligoanuria	Increased WBC
Abdominal tenderness	Petechiae	Decreased RBC
Dehydration	Jaundice	
	Change in mental status	

Abbreviations: BUN, blood urea nitrogen; RBC, red blood cell count; WBC, white blood cell count.

hemoglobin levels (5–9 g/dL), thrombocytopenia, and hemolysis on peripheral blood smear. Because of renal involvement, blood urea nitrogen (BUN) and creatinine levels are increased. Urinalysis may reveal hematuria and proteinuria, although a clean void urine sample may be difficult to obtain in children with diarrhea. Although early confirmed diagnosis of HUS is important, supportive treatment should be started as soon as there is suspicion of the diagnosis.

SUPPORTIVE CARE

Supportive treatment of HUS includes fluid management, blood product transfusions for anemia, renal replacement therapy, electrolyte replacement, and treatment of hypertension.[3] Fluid management focuses on a fine balance of maintaining renal perfusion while avoiding fluid overload. Studies have shown that, for patients with STEC/HUS, fluid administration started with early diagnosis has better short-term outcomes with fewer central nervous system (CNS) complications, and less need for renal replacement therapy and intensive care support.[10,11] Early administration of 20 mL/kg fluid bolus of isotonic crystalloid to restore intravascular volume, followed by maintenance fluids, may limit oliguria and acute renal failure.[7] Monitoring of hydration status is important, including monitoring vital signs, weight, and intake and output. When monitoring weight, it is important to remember that weight does not always indicate intravascular volume but can be a result of edema caused by vascular leakage.[11] A urinary catheter is of little value and increases risk of a hospital-acquired infection. If a patient begins to show signs of renal failure, it is important to limit fluid intake. When patients are in fluid overload when renal replacement therapy is started in critically ill children, there tends to be a poorer prognosis.[12]

Hemolysis and platelet consumption are a cause of HUS and although it may seem beneficial, platelet transfusions are contraindicated unless there is clinically significant hemorrhage or an invasive procedure is to be performed. Instead, packed red blood cell (PRBC) infusion is recommended with a reduction of hematocrit or if there is evidence of poor oxygen delivery or cardiovascular compromise. Transfusion of PRBCs is a common occurrence in patients with HUS.

Oliguria and anuria were reported in 66% of patients and dialysis therapy in 71% of patients in a study by Loos and colleagues.[13] Indications for renal replacement therapy in patients with HUS are the same as for any patient with signs of renal failure. Dialysis may be indicated for hyperkalemia (>6.5 mol/L), BUN level greater than 36 mol/L, persistent acidosis, or volume overload with cardiac or respiratory compromise.[9] Dialysis is usually required for a median range of 11 days per Loos and colleagues.[13] A correlation between an increased white blood cell count and an increased need for dialysis was confirmed.[13] A benefit has not been shown for a preference of one form of dialysis rather than another. Although it may seem like it would be a contraindication with EHEC, peritoneal dialysis has been shown to be effective for patients with HUS.

Although many of the complications of HUS are a result of renal injury, there are also extrarenal complications to be alert for. A life-threatening complication of HUS to monitor for is CNS involvement. Signs of CNS involvement include disorientation, lethargy, seizures, or coma. Encephalopathy can occur but can be decreased or avoided with the early application of dialysis.[14] Loos and colleagues[13] report severe neurologic symptoms including seizures, blurry vision, coma, decreased level of consciousness, encephalopathy, paresis, and aphasia.[13] Neurologic complications are a frequent cause of mortality. Frequent neurologic assessments should be done to monitor for life-threatening CNS involvement.

IMPLICATIONS FOR CRITICAL CARE NURSING

As discussed earlier, the care of patients with HUS is supportive, therefore nursing priorities include monitoring for disease progression, complications, implementing supportive therapies, and providing emotional support and education to the patient and family. As children in the critical care unit need close monitoring, so do patients who are admitted with HUS. Close monitoring includes vital signs, neurologic assessment, and fluid balance. Hourly vital signs, neurologic examination, and intake and output should be checked, as well as monitoring for signs of fluid volume deficit or fluid overload, depending on what clinical phase the child is in. Early in the course, while the patient may still have diarrhea and is starting with fluid resuscitation, it is important to assess for signs of dehydration, such as decreased urine output, increased heart rate, decreased skin turgor, and dry mucous membranes. If the patient has progressed to showing signs of acute kidney injury, including being oliguric or anuria, the assessment should focus on signs of fluid overload such as increased blood pressure and edema. Fluid volume status should also be monitored by weighing the patient daily. However, it is important to remember that a weight gain does not always indicate intravascular volume status; the fluid could be a result of edema with the fluid in the tissues, likely indicating kidney involvement. Neurologic examinations are important at any phase of HUS. The patient may initially present as lethargic, but hourly neurologic examinations identify decreasing neurologic function, including seizures and progression to coma.

Frequent laboratory draws are done for patients with HUS while the serum hematology and chemistry are being monitored and trended. Expected values that should be watched and reported include decreased hemoglobin level, decreased platelet count, and electrolyte changes. The most common electrolyte imbalance that can be seen indicating renal involvement is an increased potassium level. If a patient has an increased potassium level, typically more than 5.5 mmol/L, an electrocardiogram should be obtained, and the patient should be watched for arrhythmias. Because patients with HUS are already at risk for decreased hemoglobin levels secondary to the destruction of the red blood cells, it is important that nurse be aware of how much blood is sent to the laboratory. It is preferable to use Microtainers, as available, and to follow hospital policy related to readministration of blood waste for laboratory draws.

Nursing interventions focus on implementing supportive therapies such as fluid administration, red blood cell infusions, nutrition therapy, and, if there is acute kidney injury that is severe enough, renal replacement therapy such as peritoneal dialysis or continuous renal replacement therapy (CRRT). Fluid replacement depends on the clinical phase of the illness, but nurses can expect to provide maintenance fluids and replace insensible losses, and may be ordered to replace urine output milliliter for milliliter. If a patient is ordered for PRBC administration, it is important that nurses be on alert for transfusion reactions; patients who are developmentally able to understand should be taught the signs and symptoms to alert their nurses for early identification of possible reactions.

Nutritional therapy is important for patients with HUS. These children have likely experienced caloric deficits as a result of diarrhea for days, and they are ordered nothing by mouth, therefore it is important to have a nutritional consult placed early. For patients who are ordered parenteral nutrition, calorie intake should be maximized while limiting fluid volumes to prevent fluid overload.[9]

Medication administration for the patients should include pain control. However, it is important for nurses to remember that administration of nonsteroidal antiinflammatory drugs (NSAIDs) is contraindicated for patients with HUS caused by decreased renal flow.[3] Other medications of which nurses should be aware that are contraindicated for patients with HUS include antimotility agents and antibiotics.[8] Medications that nurses can expect may be ordered include furosemide and/or hypertensive agents.[9]

Care of patients with HUS who are being treated with peritoneal dialysis or CRRT is similar to that of any patient on these treatment modalities. A consideration to identify renal failure early in the disease process is that the patient may need to be transferred to another facility if a form of dialysis is needed. Parents should be aware of this possibility upfront so as to not be burdened with the additional stress of an unexpected transfer to another facility in an already stressful situation of a critically ill child.

Emotional support and education are important for patients and family/caregivers of the patients in a critical care unit with HUS. If available, a child life therapist should be consulted to help with providing developmentally appropriate activities and education for the patient. In addition, a child life therapist can provide assistance with distraction for invasive procedures that the child may experience. The family should be educated on the modes of transmission for the causative agent, STEC, and provide education as to prevention in the future. However, it is important to reassure that they are not at fault for the illness and that there is nothing they could have done to prevent the complications from the *E coli* infection.

PROGNOSIS

Most children diagnosed with HUS experience a full recovery; however, there is a risk for long-term renal sequelae. A systematic review and meta-analysis of 49 studies including children aged 1 to 18 years has shown that greater severity of illness, including dialysis, seizures, and stroke, is associated with a worse long-term prognosis.[14] However, patients who can maintain creatinine clearance greater than 80 mL min, no hypertension, and no proteinuria have an excellent long-term prognosis.[14] Additional predictors of a more severe course of illness and higher mortalities include increased white blood cell count, severe gastrointestinal prodrome, anuria early in the course of illness, and age less than 2 years. A study by Mody and colleagues[15] identified predictors of in-hospital death for patients with postdiarrheal HUS. Two of the predictors identified supported findings of previous studies, which include marked leukocytosis and higher hemoglobin and hematocrit values. The increased hemoglobin and hematocrit values are likely associated with signs of dehydration and support the administration of fluids early in the course of illness. An additional finding by Mody and colleagues[15] includes an association between recent respiratory tract infection and death following HUS. Although they do account for the fact that, for some patients in the study, pneumococcus could have been the causative agent, the other factor could be that the patient was treated with antibiotics for the respiratory tract infection. As discussed previously, antibiotics can alter intestinal flora and increase the severity of the STEC infection.

Following recovery of HUS, children benefit from long-term follow-up to identify long-term renal complications. Although the rate of long-term complications is about 30%, studies have shown that sequelae can develop as long as 10 to 15 years after HUS.[16] Long-term complications from HUS mostly affect the kidneys with hypertension, proteinuria, chronic kidney disease, and end-stage kidney disease (ESKD). Chronic kidney disease and ESKD have a higher predictability if the patient is on prolonged dialysis, 10 or more days of anuria, or did not have full recovery of renal function.[16] However, the acute mortality of HUS is low.

PREVENTION

Primary prevention for HUS is focused on prevention of EHEC infection. Good food hygiene practice helps to prevent EHEC infection. Good food hygiene practices include handwashing; keeping raw and cooked food separate; storing food at safe temperatures; and cooking food, especially ground beef, thoroughly. STEC can be destroyed by cooking food until all parts reach a temperature of 70°C or higher.[17] Prevention of secondary transmission person to person in a home or child care setting includes good hygiene practices, including handwashing.

Once diagnosed with STEC infection, there are medications that should be avoided because they have been shown to increase the risk of HUS or worsen symptoms. It has been recommended that antimotility agents be avoided. Antimotility agents prolong the *E coli* toxin in the intestine, increasing the duration of exposure to the toxin. Other medications to avoid include NSAIDs. NSAIDs increase the possibility of worsening gastrointestinal bleeding and acute renal failure, along with heparin and antithrombotic agents.[7]

SUMMARY

Pathogenic diarrhea causing *E coli* are commonly transmitted through contact with animals, persons, or contaminated water or food. Young children are at highest risk and are prone to develop a more severe illness, HUS. HUS is a clinical syndrome characterized by macroangiopathic hemolytic anemia, thrombocytopenia, and acute renal failure. Care of patients with HUS is supportive and requires early diagnosis and treatment in the acute phase of the syndrome, therefore it is essential that health care providers are alert to the symptoms of the infection and monitor closely for complications.

REFERENCES

1. Centers for Disease Control and Prevention. *E. coli* (*Escherichia coli*) 2015. Available at: https://www.cdc.gov/ecoli/general/index.html. Accessed January 17, 2017.
2. Miller VS, Levin D, Morris F, et al. Essentials of pediatric intensive care. 2nd edition. London: Churchill Livingstone; 1997.
3. DynaMed. Hemolytic-uremic syndrome 2015. Available at: http://web.b.ebscohost.com/dynamed/detail?vid=4&sid=f47bc3c9-2edc-4b63-99e8-1d502df5d2db%40sessionmgr101&bdata=JnNpdGU9ZHluYW1lZC1saXZlJnNjb3BlPXNpdGU%3d#anchor=References&AN=116202&db=dme. Accessed January 17, 2017.

4. Cieślik P, Bartoszcze M. Enterohaemorrhagic *Escherichia coli* (EHEC) infections: a threat to public health. Med Weter 2011;67(9):571–8.

5. Centers for Disease Control and Prevention (CDC). Multistate outbreak of Shiga toxin-producing *Escherichia coli* O157:H7 infections linked to I.M. Healthy brand SoyNut butter (final update). In *E. coli (Escherichia coli)* 2017. Available at: https://www.cdc.gov/ecoli/2017/o157h7-03-17/index.html. Accessed June 6, 2017.

6. Wong CS, Mooney JC, Brandt JR, et al. Risk factors for the hemolytic uremic syndrome in children infected with *Escherichia coli* O157: H7: a multivariable analysis. Clin Infect Dis 2012;55(1):33–41.

7. Mele C, Remuzzi G, Noris M. Hemolytic uremic syndrome. Semin Immunopathol 2014;36(4):399–420.

8. Freedman S, Xie J, Neufeld M, et al. Shiga toxin-producing *Escherichia coli* infection, antibiotics, and risk of developing hemolytic uremic syndrome: a meta-analysis. Clin Infect Dis 2016;62(10):1251–8.

9. Hazinski M. Renal disorders. In: Nursing care of the critically ill child. 3rd edition. St Louis (MO): Elsevier; 2013. p. 703–69.

10. Ardissino G, Tel F, Possenti I, et al. Early volume expansion and outcomes of hemolytic uremic syndrome. Pediatrics 2015;137(1):e20152153.

11. Balestracci A, Sandra M, Toledo I, et al. Dehydration at admission increased the need for dialysis in hemolytic uremic syndrome children. Pediatr Nephrol 2012; 27:1407–10.

12. Goldstein SL, Somers MJ, Baum MA, et al. Pediatric patients with multiorgan dysfunction syndrome receiving continuous renal replacement therapy. Kidney Int 2005;67(2):653–8.

13. Loos S, Ahlenstiel T, Kranz B, et al. An outbreak of Shiga toxin–producing *Escherichia coli* O104: H4 hemolytic uremic syndrome in Germany: presentation and short-term outcome in children. Clin Infect Dis 2012;55(6):753–9.

14. Garg AX, Suri RS, Barrowman N, et al. Long-term renal prognosis of diarrhea-associated hemolytic uremic syndrome: a systematic review, meta-analysis, and meta-regression. JAMA 2003;290(10):1360–70.

15. Mody R, Weidong G, Griffin P, et al. Postdiarrheal hemolytic uremic syndrome in Unites States children: clinical spectrum and predictors of in-hospital death. J Pediatr 2015;166(4):1022–9.

16. Spinale J, Ruebner R, Copelovitch L, et al. Long-term outcomes of Shiga toxin hemolytic uremic syndrome. Pediatr Nephrol 2013;28:2097–105.

17. World Health Organization. E. coli. 2016. Available at: http://www.who.int/mediacentre/factsheets/fs125/en/. Accessed February 6, 2017.

Gastrointestinal Traumatic Injuries

Gastrointestinal Perforation

Maria A. Revell, PhD, RN, MSN, COI[a],*,
Marcia A. Pugh, DNP, RN, MBA, HCM, MSN[b],
Melanie McGhee, MSN, RN, ACNP-BC[c]

KEYWORDS

- Gastrointestinal trauma • Trauma • Hemorrhagic shock • OPQRST • SAMPLE

KEY POINTS

- Gastrointestinal trauma can result in injury to the stomach, small bowel, colon, or rectum. Anatomic abdominal organ placement can determine the potential of injury for nontraumatic and traumatic injury.
- Motor vehicle accidents can result in seatbelt-associated injuries collectively called "the seatbelt syndrome" which has been validated as indicative of an increased risk of gastrointestinal injury.
- Gastrointestinal penetrating wounds include those caused by low- or high-velocity actions which result in varying management based on accompanying injuries and institutional resources.
- Use of the Penetrating Abdominal Trauma Index can assist health care providers in validation of severity for patients with penetrating abdominal wounds.

INTRODUCTION

The abdomen is a big place even in a small person. Numerous systems are housed in the abdomen and directly affect the gastrointestinal system. These systems include the (a) integumentary system, (b) cardiovascular system, (c) neurologic system, (d) urologic system, (d) gynecologic system, and (e) orthopedic system, to name a few.

Disclosure Statement: The authors have no financial interests, affiliations, or conflicts of interest that relate to the publication of this material.
[a] School of Nursing, Tennessee State University, 3500 John A Merritt Boulevard, Campus Box 9590, Nashville, TN 37132, USA; [b] Grants, Research and Outreach of West AL Division, Tombigbee Healthcare Authority, 105 US Highway 80 East, Demopolis, AL 36732, USA; [c] Department of Structural Heart, St. Thomas West Hospital, 4330 Harding Road, Suite 535, Nashville, TN 37205, USA
* Corresponding author.
E-mail address: mrevell1@tnstate.edu

The gastrointestinal traumatic injury of gastrointestinal perforation can come from disease that originates in other systems and invades the gastrointestinal system. Perforation of the esophagus, stomach, small intestine, large intestine, or rectum can result from a variety of causes that are traumatic or nontraumatic. Traumatic causes include blunt or penetrating trauma, such as gunshot wounds, stabbings, motor vehicle collisions (MVCs), and crush injuries. Nontraumatic causes include appendicitis, Crohn disease, cancer, diverticulitis, ulcerative colitis, blockage of the bowel, and chemotherapy.

Gastrointestinal trauma can result in injury to the stomach, small bowel, colon, or rectum. This trauma can occur from blunt or penetrating injuries. The mechanism of injury will affect both the nature and the severity of any resulting injuries. MVC seatbelt restraint use accounts for approximately 75% of gastrointestinal trauma with potential perforation. Seatbelt placement is implicated in this trauma category.[1]

Gastrointestinal Organs

The anatomic placement of abdominal organs can determine injury potential. The stomach is located in the left upper abdominal quadrant. Anatomically, it is located adjacent to the diaphragm, liver, colon, and abdominal wall anteriorly. Structures that are posterior to the stomach include the left kidney and adrenal gland, spleen, splenic artery, pancreas, transverse colon, megacolon, and left diaphragm. The gastric arteries provide blood supply to the stomach.

The small bowel is anatomically divided into 3 distinct portions. These portions are the duodenum, jejunum, and ileum. The duodenum is predominantly retroperitoneal. The duodenum consists of 4 segments, an initial one of which is transverse. This first segment starts at the pylorus and ends at the common bile duct superiorly and gastroduodenal artery inferiorly. A second segment is inferior to the ampulla of Vater. A third segment is transverse to the superior mesenteric vein and artery. A fourth portion extends from where the duodenum emerges from the retroperitoneum and joins the jejunum. A large portion of the duodenum lies directly over the spinal column. The duodenum arterial supply arrives from the celiac artery. There is additional circulatory support from the right gastric artery. Venous drainage follows arterial pathways.

The colon and rectum also occupy gastrointestinal space. The colon structures are transverse, ascending, and descending. The transverse colon is intraperitoneal and extends from the hepatic flexure to the splenic flexure. The ascending and descending colons are retroperitoneal. The rectum measures 12 to 15 cm and continues distally from the colon. The rectum is anterior to several bony structures. They are the sacral vertebrae and coccyx. It is posterior to the vagina in women and the bladder in men.

Trauma

Many gastrointestinal injuries result from MVCs. These injuries can occur from a vehicular collision with another vehicle, an animal, road debris, a pedestrian, or a stationary object (eg, utility pole, building, tree, roadway abutment). Airborne vehicle accidents can produce the same type of injuries caused by MVCs depending on the object of impact upon landing. Other causes of gastrointestinal injury include penetrating wounds that can occur from knife or other sharp penetrating object injuries and gunshot wounds. They can even occur from seatbelt use, especially those that fit across the pelvic area.

Seatbelt syndrome

Seatbelts are designed to keep occupants from being thrown from or within the vehicle upon impact. Seatbelt nonuse has been associated with several significant factors, including male sex, young age, passenger versus driver, risk-taking behaviors, living in a rural setting, having few dependents, smoking, speeding, alcohol consumption, low educational level, black or Hispanic ethnicity, or traveling on secondary versus primary roadways.[2] Their purpose is to prevent the driver from coming in contact with the steering wheel and front seat occupants from contacting the dashboard and windshield. Seatbelts significantly reduce trauma to the head, face, chest, abdomen, and extremities.[3] Although there are benefits to wearing seatbelts, there are potential injuries that can result.[4] There is increasing reported injury of gastrointestinal trauma from seatbelts. Injury results from the redistribution of forces that occur during impact. The collective term used for seatbelt-associated injuries is called "the seatbelt syndrome."[5] This seatbelt syndrome is most often associated with use of a lap belt and identified by a bruising pattern that follows the course of the seatbelt itself across an individual's torso.[6] The seatbelt sign has been validated as indicative of an increased risk of gastrointestinal injury.[7,8]

The spectrum of injuries from seatbelt injuries includes not only gastrointestinal injuries but also bony injuries. Gastrointestinal injuries include mesenteric tears, hollow visceral blowouts, and abdominal and solid organ contusions.[2] Injury to bony structures can include fractures and dislocations of the spine. These injuries occur from rapid deceleration of abdominal structures because they are held in place during impact.

Intervention involves early detection of intra-abdominal bleeding through assessment and laboratory and radiologic evaluation. Some signs that may indicate seatbelt syndrome include increasing abdominal tenderness and/or bruising. There may also be an abrasion across the lower abdomen from the seatbelt. Management of seatbelt syndrome involves early diagnosis and intervention. Evaluation should include history and thorough assessment noting current conditions of the external abdominal wall and continued evaluation to observe for occurring changes (eg, ecchymosis). Diagnostic tests include imaging for validation. Surgical intervention may or may not be necessary.

Traumatic abdominal wall hernia

Gastrointestinal injury can include an acute traumatic abdominal wall hernia (TAWH). This type of herniation injury can occur from high impact or low impact to the abdominal wall. High-energy injuries can occur during MVCs or vehicle versus pedestrian accidents. Low-energy herniations can occur as a result of abdominal wall impact on a small (focused) blunt object.[9,10] In a TAWH injury, the abdominal wall comes in contact with a blunt object that is focused in its intensity. Abdominal wall herniation can be associated with a high percent of intra-abdominal injuries.[11] In 50 cases examined in the English literature, 69% were small bowel, 36% were large bowel, and 16% contained injuries to both bowel sections. Because of its uncommon presentation of approximately 1% of blunt trauma admissions,[12] up to 20% of TAWH injuries can go unrecognized, but based on evidence, immediate surgical intervention is supported.[13]

TAWH occurs when there is perforation of the abdominal viscera with an intact outer abdominal wall. This type of injury is also referred to as a "handlebar hernia." This type of injury has been reported to occur with various types of accidents (**Box 1**). TAWH can present as ecchymosis and/or a localized palpable hernia. An area of ecchymosis can surround the hernia and develop soon after the initial accident. Any quadrant of the abdomen can be involved (right upper, right lower, left upper, or left lower). The herniation can contain abdominal contents, such as the small bowel, transverse colon, ileum, sigmoid colon, or cecum.

Management of a TAWH involves early diagnosis and intervention (**Fig. 1**). Evaluation should include history and thorough assessment, noting current conditions of the external abdominal wall and continued evaluation to observe for occurring changes (eg, ecchymosis and/or bulges). Diagnostic tests include imaging for validation of herniation presence and degree of involvement of gastrointestinal contents. With confirmed or highly suspected diagnosis of TAWH, surgical intervention can include laparotomy or laparoscopy. This intervention can vary by hernia location. The highest report of acute therapeutic surgical intervention occurred with anterior abdominal hernias.[11]

Penetrating gastrointestinal injuries

Penetrating wounds include those caused by low- or high-velocity actions. Severity depends on the mechanism of injury. These wounds can be caused by foreign instruments, hand guns or long guns, and archery bows. Management varies based on injury mechanism and location, hemodynamic stability, neurologic status, associated injuries that accompany the gastrointestinal trauma, and institutional resources. Routine laparotomy can be one response to penetrating wound management. Nonoperative management of penetrating abdominal wounds was addressed by the Shaftan report.[14] This report identified that of the 92% of patients studied with stab wounds operative intervention was initiated if the patient had primary peritoneal irritation manifested by abdominal tenderness, rebound tenderness, reduced or absent bowel sounds or secondary signs of blood per rectum, positive paracentesis, or hematemesis. There was no mortality in patients with nonoperative treatment.[14] Selective observation can be a safe method to patient management (**Fig. 2**).[15] Patients who have experienced stab wounds who are hemodynamically stable without signs of peritonitis or diffuse tenderness of the abdomen do not require routine laparotomy. Routine laparotomy is also not indicated in patients with tangential abdominal gunshot wounds without peritoneal signs.[14]

Nursing management

Historical information is important to retrieve. Emergency medical services are often initially on the scene and able to relay key information to receiving organizations upon transport. Transmission of key information can be crucial in situations where

---

Box 1
Mechanisms of injury that can cause traumatic abdominal wall hernia

1. MCA handlebar trauma

2. MVC restrained and unrestrained passenger

3. Compression injury occurring when individual caught between motor vehicle and stationary object

4. Fall from a height onto a blunt object

5. Pedestrian struck by motor vehicle

6. Bicycle handlebar

7. Blunt trauma from collapsed building structures

Abbreviations: MCA, motor cycle accident; MVC, motor vehicle collision.

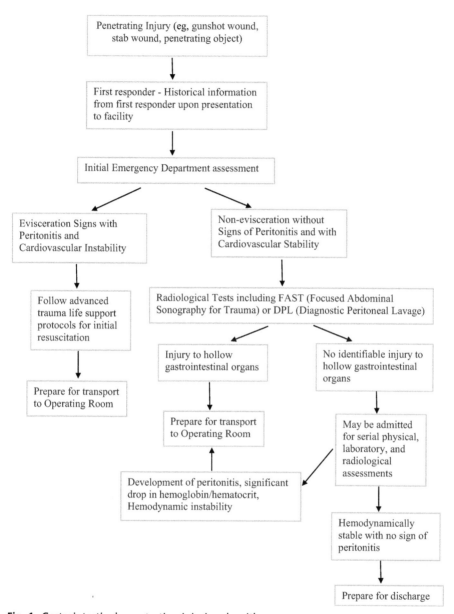

Fig. 1. Gastrointestinal penetrating injuries algorithm.

the patient is critically ill or has an altered mental status. Acronyms can be used to solicit data collection in an organized technique. Some of the more common acronyms are listed.

AMPLE
- Allergies
- Medications
- Prior illnesses and operations

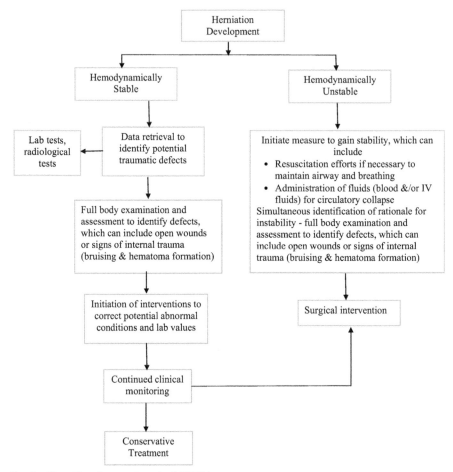

Fig. 2. Algorithm for treatment of TAWH.

- Last meal
- Events and environment surrounding injury[16]

SAMPLE

- Signs and symptoms
- Allergies
- Medications
- Past medical history or pertinent history
- Last oral intake
- Events leading to incident/injury[17]

OPQRST

- Onset of event
- Provocation or palliation
- Quality of pain
- Region or radiation
- Severity
- Time (history)[18]

Injury location, type of weapon or object that caused penetration, and position of the person during injury all facilitate identification of current and future care techniques. The number of penetrations is also taken into consideration. Close-range injuries transfer more kinetic energy; however, gunshot wounds may be difficult to determine closeness and velocity.[16] Aggressive fluid resuscitation is not recommended prehospital in order to maintain normotension unless the injured individual manifests severe shock. Fluid may be necessary if transport time is extended or to maintain mentation status.[16]

Use of the Penetrating Abdominal Trauma Index (PATI) can assist in validation of severity for patients with penetrating abdominal wounds. Each organ is given a score with a range from 1 to 5 (**Table 1**). The percent injury to an organ can indicate how much the entire circumference is involved with resulting injury. An organ score is calculated by multiplying the injury estimate by the risk factor. For example, the stomach has a risk factor of 2, whereas the large intestine has a risk factor of 4. If injury involves the colon wall and blood supply, the injury estimate is 5. The organ score for the large intestine would be 20. The overall index has a score range from 0 to 200. Risk of

Table 1 Penetrating Abdominal Trauma Index		
Organ/Site of Injury	**Risk Factor from Highest to Lowest**	**Severity Grade Range of Injury Range**
Duodenum	5	Single wall damage = 1 to surgical pancreatic duodenectomy required for intervention = 5
Pancreas	5	Tangential damage = 1 to pancreatic duodenectomy required for intervention = 5
Liver	4	Nonbleeding peripheral damage = 1 to lobectomy with caval repair or debridement (extensive bilobar) required
Large Intestine	4	Serous intestinal layer damage = 1 to damage to the colon wall as well as the blood supply = 5
Major Vascular	4	≤25% wall damage = 1 to ligation required = 5
Spleen	3	Nonbleeding damage = 1 to splenectomy required for intervention = 5
Kidney	3	Nonbleeding injury = 1 to nephrectomy required for intervention = 5
Extrahepatic biliary	2	Contusion injury = 1 to biliary reconstruction = 5
Small Bowel	2	Single wall damage = 1 to wall structural and blood supply damage = 5
Stomach	2	Single wall damage = 1 to stomach resection required for intervention = 5
Ureter	2	Contusion injury = 1 to ureter reconstruction required for intervention = 5
Bladder	1	Single wall injury = 1 to bladder reconstruction required for intervention = 5
Bone	1	Periosteum damage = 1 to major bone loss = 5
Minor Vascular	1	Nonbleeding vessel damage = 1 to required ligation of vessels = 5

Data from Refs.[24–27]

postoperative complications is low if the PATI is equal to or less than 25% and sharply increases if the PATI is greater than 25%.

Gastrointestinal bleeding can range from minor loss to massive hemorrhage. Major vessels that support gastrointestinal organs and the lower extremities go through the abdomen. These vessels are increased in size to move large quantities of oxygenated and unoxygenated blood. Perforating instruments can significantly damage arterial and venous vessels, causing considerable blood loss and subsequent shock if not addressed. The primary treatment of hemorrhagic shock caused by blood loss is identification and repair of the defect causing the loss.

Blood loss can cause various patterns on the abdominal wall over time. The Cullen sign is bruising around the umbilicus. It can indicate hemoperitoneum or retroperitoneal bleeding. A Grey Turner sign may indicate retroperitoneal bleeding. Both of these signs can take up to 12 hours or more to appear, so initial evaluation needs to be followed with intermittent evaluation over time. Intermittent evaluation is necessary because slow bleeding from the abdominal viscera or other internal organs may not be clinically apparent until a significant amount of blood has accumulated in the abdominal cavity. Based on the care provider's index of suspicion for hypovolemia, additional radiographic testing may be done to validate or rule out bleeding. Persistent tachycardia can be used to identify continued tissue hypoxia, which needs to be addressed. A pulse greater than 100 beats per minute can indicate blood loss of 1500 to 2000 mL. A pulse greater than 140 beats per minute can indicate blood loss in excess of 2000 mL.[19] Pulse pressure can correlate with the volume of blood ejected from the left ventricle. It can be used as an indication of vascular bed volume. Management of hypovolemia and anemia requires immediate volume resuscitation with balanced salt solutions and blood products.

Penetrating abdominal objects may invade gastrointestinal organs. Management of penetrating object trauma is important. If an individual is impaled, they may appear in the acute care facility emergency department with part of the object intact but secured by emergency medical personnel. The position of these objects is not to be altered by nursing personnel and never removed outside of a surgical suite because removal could result in additional injury. The patient is to have immediate surgical preparation whereby the object can be removed under controlled circumstances. If evisceration of gastrointestinal organs is present due to an abdominal traumatic opening (eg, knife wound with intestinal evisceration), the contents should be covered with a saline-soaked gauze and a sterile towel until surgical evaluation has been completed.[19]

Pain management of patients with gastrointestinal injuries is important but must be undertaken with extreme caution. Pain can indicate the severity of an injury so serves a positive purpose. On the negative side, it can cause additional complications, such as increase heart rate and blood pressure, which further increases oxygen needs and consumption. It is important to be aware of the fact that an individual who has experienced severe trauma is anxious and may still be fearful as a result of the traumatic incident.[20] The nurse must carefully assess pain and use age-appropriate scales. In order to provide optimum pain management, nurses must be familiar with age-specific pharmacologic management as well as the adverse effects of pain management. It is important to not withhold ordered medication for fear of addiction or the patient's history of past narcotic use. Pain medication given at appropriate intervals and in response to request for medicinal intervention can reduce the stress response, promote healing, shorten the hospital stay, lower health care costs, and reduce morbidity and mortality.[21] The World Health Organization recommends pain medication be given on a clock schedule of every 3 to 6 hours. Their medicinal pain relief ladder includes the 3 following steps: (a) nonopioid medication, (b), opioid for mild to moderate pain plus or minus nonopioid medications and if pain persists or increases, (c) opioid for moderate to severe pain, plus or minus nonopioid medications.[22,23] Providing appropriate and timely medication for pain management improves patient outcomes. It increases satisfaction with care as well.

SUMMARY

Prudent judgment is necessary in management of the patient with gastrointestinal injuries whether they result in open abdominal wounds or not. Assessment starts in the field and continues in the acute care setting. In order to promote the best possible outcome, the nurse must respond quickly and be familiar with potential outcomes that promote successful recovery. This knowledge promotes movement of the patient in the direction of management components that facilitate a positive outcome. Pain management is important, but medication must be given with caution in order to reduce the potential for respiratory and/or cardiovascular instability. Pain medication can also mask abdominal pain whereby pain can be a sign and symptom of intervention urgency. Knowledge of both surgical and nonsurgical interventions is important to note in order to prepare the patient for either potential surgical or nonsurgical interventions and educate them regarding postintervention self-care.

REFERENCES

1. Isenhour JL, Marx J. Advances in abdominal trauma. Emerg Med Clin North Am 2007;25(3):713–33.
2. Intas G, Stergiannis P. Seat belt syndrome: a global issue. Health Sci J 2010;4(4): 202–9.
3. Orsay EM, Dunne M, Turnbull TL, et al. Prospective study of the effect of seatbelts in motor vehicle crashes. Ann Emerg Med 1990;19:258–61.
4. Hamilton JB. Seat-belt injuries. Br Med J 1968;4(5629):485–6.
5. Al-Ozaibi L, Adnan J, Hassan B, et al. Seat belt syndrome: delayed or missed intestinal injuries, a case report and review of literature. Int J Surg Case Rep 2016. https://doi.org/10.1016/j.ijscr.2016.01.015.
6. Doersch KB, Dozier WE. The seat belt sign, intestinal and mesenteric injuries. Am J Surg 1968;116(6):831–3.
7. Wotherspoon S, Chu K, Brown AF, et al. Abdominal injury and the seat-belt sign. Emerg Med (Fremantle) 2001;13(1):61–5.
8. Cornelissen MP, van Buijtenen J, van den Heuvel B, et al. Blunt abdominal wall disruption by seatbelt injury; a case report and review of the literature. Bull Emerg Trauma 2016;4(2):105–9.
9. Lane CT, Cohen AJ, Cinat ME, et al. Management of traumatic abdominal wall hernia. Am Surg 2003;69(1):73–6.
10. Hamidian Jahromi A, Skweres J, Sangster G, et al. What we know about management of traumatic abdominal wall hernia: review of the literature and case report. Int Surg 2015;100(2):233–9.
11. Coleman JJ, Fitz EK, Zarzaur BL, et al. Traumatic abdominal wall hernias: location matters. J Trauma Acute Care Surg 2016;80(3):380–6.
12. Pardhan A, Mazahir S, Rao S, et al. Blunt traumatic abdominal wall hernias: a surgeon's dilemma. World J Surg 2015;40(1):231–5.
13. Suhardja TS, Atalla MA, Rozen WM. Complete abdominal wall disruption with herniation following blunt injury: case report and review of the literature. Int Surg 2015;100(3):531–9.

14. Como JJ, Bokhari F, Chiu WC, et al. Practice management guidelines for selective nonoperative management of penetrating abdominal trauma. J Trauma 2010; 68(3):721–33.
15. Arikan S, Kocakusak A, Yucel AF, et al. A prospective comparison of the selective observation and routine exploration methods for penetrating abdominal stab wounds with organ or omentum evisceration. J Trauma 2005;58(3):526–32.
16. Offner P. Penetrating abdominal trauma clinical presentation. Medscape 2017. Available at: http://emedicine.medscape.com/article/2036859-clinical.
17. Understanding the SAMPLE History. The EMT Spot. 2012. Available at: http://theemtspot.com/2012/03/08/understanding-the-sample-history/.
18. Friese G. How to use OPQRST as an effective patient assessment tool. EMS1.com 3 2010. Available at: https://www.ems1.com/ems-products/education/tips/475522-How-to-use- OPQRST-as-an-effective-patient-assessment-tool/.
19. Saunorus M, Bethel S. Manual of critical care nursing: nursing interventions and collaborative management. 6th edition. St. Louis (MO): Elsevier; 2010.
20. Ahmadi A, Bazargan-Hejazi S, Heidari Zadie Z, et al. Pain management in trauma: a review study. J Inj Violence Res 2016;8(2):89–98.
21. Malchow RJ, Black IH. The evolution of pain management in the critically ill trauma patient: emerging concepts from the global war on terrorism. Crit Care Med 2008;36(7 Suppl):S346–57.
22. WHO's Pain Relief Ladder. World Health Organization. 2017. Available at: http://www.who.int/cancer/palliative/painladder/en/. Accessed January 12, 2017.
23. Penetrating Abdominal Trauma Index (PATI). Medal military medicine. 2017. Available at: http://www.medal.org/. Accessed April 14, 2017.
24. Moore EE, Dunn EL, Moore JB, et al. Penetrating abdominal trauma index. J Trauma 1981;21(6):439–45.
25. Gomez-Leon JF. Penetrating abdominal trauma index: Sensitivity and specificity for morbidity and mortality by ROC analysis. Indian J Surg 2004;66:347–51.
26. Naqvi S, Effendi S, Zafar H. High PATI score is associated with increase mortality in patients with penetrating abdominal injuries; a retrospective review. Nat J Health Sci 2016;1(1):30–3. Available at: http://ecommons.aku.edu/pakistan_fhs_mc_surg_gen/30. Accessed October 31, 2017.
27. Penetrating Abdominal Trauma Index (PATI). Available at: https://www.medicalalgorithms.com/penetrating-abdominal-trauma-index-pati. Accessed October 31, 2017.

Gastroesophageal Reflux

Regurgitation in the Infant Population

Teresa D. Ferguson, DNP, RN, CNE[a,b,*]

KEYWORDS

- Gastroesophageal reflux • Gastroesophageal reflux disease • Infants
- Growth failure • Treatment

KEY POINTS

- Gastroesophageal reflux (GER) is common disorder in infants.
- This condition can become acute with infants developing symptoms of gastroesophageal reflux disease (GERD), which includes poor weight gain, continued irritability, abnormal posturing, and respiratory complications.
- Infants presenting with symptoms of GERD should be immediately referred to a pediatric specialist to treat and prevent further complications.

Gastroesophageal reflux (GER) is common disorder in infants through 12 months of age.[1] This condition can become acute with infants developing symptoms of gastroesophageal reflux disease (GERD), which includes poor weight gain, continued irritability, abnormal posturing, and respiratory complications. Infants presenting with these symptoms should be immediately referred to a pediatric specialist to treat and prevent further complications.

GASTROESOPHAGEAL REFLUX
Definition

GER is the natural movement of gastric contents from the stomach into the esophagus or mouth, which may be swallowed or regurgitated.[2,3] Regurgitation may occur after feedings more than 6 times per day in some infants.[4]

Occurrence in the Infant Population

Many infants experience several episodes of GER during a 24-hour period without any adverse effects over the first few months of life.[2] GER is present in over three-fourths

---

Disclosure Statement: No conflicts of interest exist.
[a] Department of Nursing, Morehead State University, 201M Center for Health, Education and Research, 316 West Second Street, Morehead, KY 40351, USA; [b] Woman's Care Unit, St. Claire HealthCare, 222 Medical Circle, Morehead, KY 40351, USA
* Department of Nursing, Morehead State University, 201M Center for Health, Education and Research, 316 West Second Street, Morehead, KY 40351.
E-mail address: t.ferguson@moreheadstate.edu

Crit Care Nurs Clin N Am 30 (2018) 167–177
https://doi.org/10.1016/j.cnc.2017.10.015
0899-5885/18/© 2017 Elsevier Inc. All rights reserved.

of the infant population and appears in boys approximately 2 times more often than girls.[5] Infants may begin having GER before 2 months of age.[4]

Clinical Features/Symptoms

The most common clinical feature of GER in infants is postprandial regurgitation, which will often go away around 12 months of age without any treatment.[2,3] The episodes of reflux will often decrease in occurrence as the infant approaches 1 year of age.[4] Usually the infant will have no apparent symptoms other than uncomplicated spitting up and will appear comfortable and show adequate weight gain.[6]

Treatment of Gastroesophageal Reflux

The American Academy of Pediatrics recommends that providers follow the Pediatric Gastroesophageal Reflux Clinical Practice Guidelines, which are joint recommendations of the North American Society of Pediatric Gastroenterology, Hepatology, and Nutrition (NASPGHAN) and the European Society for Pediatric Gastroenterology, Hepatology, and Nutrition (ESPGHAN) in evaluation and management GER and GERD.[7] These guidelines include

- Evidence-based clinical pathways that practitioners may use as a guide with infants and children who present with GER
- Diagnostic process of GER/GERD including performing the history and physical examination
- Diagnostic studies used to identify reflux and/or complications
- Treatment including lifestyle modifications (adjustments to feeding and positioning), use of medication, and surgical procedures with GERD[3]

The newborn period is sometimes a stressful time for new parents who are trying to adjust to parenthood and meet the needs of their newborn babies. Nurses may alleviate some stress of the parents by educating them about regurgitation prior to their infant's discharge from the hospital. They will need to be taught about breastfeeding or how to properly prepare formula, how much and how often to feed the baby and oropharyngeal suctioning with a bulb syringe. It is important to instruct parents on what to do if their infant has episodes of regurgitation after hospital discharge and when to call their health care provider or return to the hospital for problems. It is also important to teach parents how to position their babies after eating and while sleeping.

Parents often seek medical help or inquire about regurgitation during follow-up visits with their health care provider. Approximately 25% of pediatric appointments are associated with complaints of GER during the first 6 months after birth.[8] Health care providers reinforce that this a normal occurrence up to 1 year of age and should provide continual reassurance to new parents.

If parents seek medical advice regarding excessive regurgitation or spitting up, health care providers need to be aware of evidence-based clinical practice guidelines related to the diagnosis and treatment of GER/GERD. The joint recommendations of the NASPGHAN and ESPGHAN include clinical pathways for health care providers to use as a guide for diagnosis and treatment of recurrent regurgitation and vomiting (**Fig. 1**).[3] The health care provider will need to obtain an accurate history and perform a physical examination of the infant, observing for clinical manifestations related to GER. If there are not any warning signs (**Box 1**) that may indicate any other type of diagnosis or signs of complicated GERD, the health care provider may conclude that uncomplicated GER is the issue, and no further testing is necessary.[3]

The treatment approach for GER involves giving support and guidance to parents along with education about lifestyle modifications for the infant such as adjustments to feeding and positioning. Providers need to reassure parents that GER is a common issue experienced by many infants during the first year of life and will resolve on its own.[3,8,9] Parents need to be given the warning signs (see **Box 1**) associated with complications that need to be reported to the health care provider when exhibited by their infants.[3] These warning signs may indicate that the infant has GERD or another health care problem that needs immediate referral for medical treatment.

Lifestyle modifications may reduce the incidence of GER, which include switching the infant's formula to another type, decreasing the amount of intake during each feeding, and increasing the number of feedings throughout the day.[8] Feeding infants excessive amounts of formula or breastmilk may increase the frequency of spitting up.[3] Therefore, it may be beneficial to decrease the amount per feeding. In order to maintain the appropriate number of calories, it may be necessary to increase the frequency of feedings throughout the day.[3] Infants need to have an accurate assessment of how many calories are required for them per feeding to ensure that enough calories for appropriate weight gain are consumed during feedings.[4]

A cow's milk protein allergy may cause increased regurgitation in infants, which closely resembles GERD.[3,4] Regurgitation may resolve or decrease in frequency by changing the formula to a noncow's milk protein-based formula (**Box 2**) or instructing breastfeeding moms to eliminate milk from their diet for a short period of time.[3,4]

Another approach is the use of thickened formulas to eliminate or decrease the episodes of spitting up.[3,8] One study found that the use of thickened feedings with carob bean gum was beneficial in decreasing the number and volume of regurgitation experienced by infants with uncomplicated GER.[10] When rice cereal is used to thicken formula, the energy density increases from 20-kcal/ounce to 34 or 27-kcal/ounce depending on whether 1 tablespoon of rice per one (1) or two (2) ounces of formula is used.[3]

It is recommended to keep infants positioned upright for at least 20 minutes after a feeding to decrease episodes of regurgitation.[11] Studies showed that infants had less reflux when positioned prone after feedings.[3] However, infants need to be positioned on their backs during sleep to decrease the risk of sudden infant death syndrome (SIDS). The excessive regurgitation should go away by one and a half years of age with uncomplicated GER. If it continues, a referral for further evaluation by a pediatric gastroenterologist is indicated.[3] The literature does not provide evidence in support of using antisecretory or promotility medications to treat uncomplicated GER.[3,4] Refer to the case study provided in **Box 3** and answers in **Box 4**.

MANAGEMENT OF CHRONIC REGURGITATION/VOMITING

Management of chronic regurgitation/vomiting begins with obtaining a history and physical examination to identify which signs and symptoms are present, rule out other conditions, and determine if problems associated with GERD are present.[3] Immediate assessment is needed to avoid the infant becoming seriously ill. For example, an infant with excessive vomiting may become dehydrated and experience a fluid and electrolyte imbalance if left untreated. Immediate interventions may prevent the infant from becoming unstable or critically ill. It may not be possible to diagnose GERD on signs and symptoms alone in infants, and further testing may be performed to confirm the diagnosis.[3] GERD is suspected when the testing indicates frequent occurrence of reflux events, esophagitis, or other diagnoses have not been established based on the signs and symptoms exhibited with the frequent

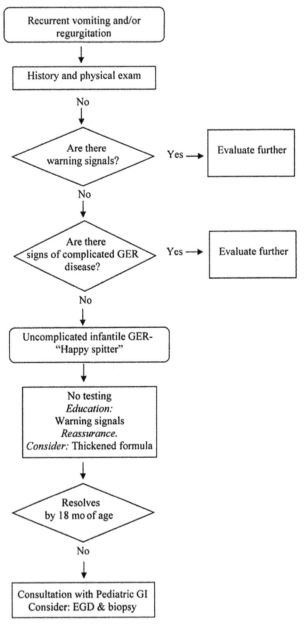

Fig. 1. Approach to the infant with recurrent regurgitation and vomiting. (*From* European Society for Pediatric Gastroenterology, Hepatology, and Nutrition and North American Society for Pediatric Gastroenterology, Hepatology, and Nutrition. Pediatric gastroesophageal reflux clinical practice guidelines: joint recommendations of the North America Society for Pediatric Gastroenterology, Hepatology, and Nutrition (NASPGHAN) and the European Society for Pediatric Gastroenterology, Hepatology, and Nutrition (ESPGHAN). J Pediatr Gastroenterol Nutr 2009;49:519; with permission.)

Box 1
Warning signs requiring investigation in infants with regurgitation or vomiting

Bilious vomiting

GI bleeding
  Hematemesis
  Hematochezia

Consistently forceful vomiting

Onset of vomiting after 6 months of life

Failure to thrive

Diarrhea

Constipation

Fever

Lethargy

Hepatosplenomegaly

Bulging fontanelle

Macro/microcephaly

Seizures

Abdominal tenderness or distension

Documented or suspected genetic/metabolic syndrome

From European Society for Pediatric Gastroenterology, Hepatology, and Nutrition and North American Society for Pediatric Gastroenterology, Hepatology, and Nutrition. Pediatric gastroesophageal reflux clinical practice guidelines: joint recommendations of the North America Society for Pediatric Gastroenterology, Hepatology, and Nutrition (NASPGHAN) and the European Society for Pediatric Gastroenterology, Hepatology, and Nutrition (ESPGHAN). J Pediatr Gastroenterol Nutr 2009;49:506; with permission.

---

occurrence of reflux. Several tests have been beneficial in confirming GERD, determining the effectiveness of therapy, or ruling out other problems.[3] Some of the tests ordered to assist in diagnosis of GERD or ruling out other disorders are intraluminal esophageal pH monitoring, multiple intraluminal impedance, motility studies, upper gastrointestinal (GI) endoscopy and biopsy, upper GI series, nuclear scintigraphy, and testing on ear, lung and esophageal fluids.[3]

GASTROESOPHAGEAL REFLUX DISEASE
Definition

GERD is the movement of gastric contents from the stomach into the esophagus or mouth, which results in some kind of pathologic problem.[3] If problems are associated with the GER such as poor weight gain, continued irritability, and respiratory problems, GERD is suspected, and further evaluation is needed.[2,3]

Occurrence in the Infant Population

Approximately one-fourth of infants in Western Europe and North America are diagnosed with GERD, which is significantly less than the prevalence of GER.[7] The incidence of severe-chronic GERD is higher in infants who are born prematurely or suffer from neurologic injury (ie, cerebral palsy) and chronic respiratory conditions.[3]

Box 2
Cow's milk protein allergy options for formula

Amino acid-based

Hydrolyzed

Soy

Data from American Academy of Pediatrics. Ages and stages: choosing a formula. Healthychildre-n.org Web site. Published 2009. Updated November 21, 2015. Available at: https://healthychildren. org/English/ages-stages/baby/feeding-nutrition/Pages/Choosing-a-Formula.aspx. Accessed June 27, 2017.

Clinical Features/Symptoms

The clinical symptoms associated with GERD include repeated regurgitation espe-cially after feedings, failure to gain weight, irritability, feeding problems, episodes of ceasing to breathe for greater than 20 seconds, or respiratory complications.[1] Infants may also have recurring episodes of pneumonia resulting from aspiration of stomach contents and issues with posturing such as arching of the back.[1] It is important to refer infants to the hospital for further evaluation by a pediatric specialist including a possible upper gastrointestinal (GI) endoscopy and biopsies with the presence of any of the warning signs (see **Box 1**) associated with complications.[4]

Treatment of Gastroesophageal Reflux Disease

The treatment for GERD is more extensive than that of GER. Quitadamo and col-leagues found that the NASPGHAN-ESPGHAN clinical practice guidelines are under-used by Italian pediatricians when treating children with GERD, indicating the need for increased education with providers directed at the correct use of the guidelines. The 3 options for managing the care of infants experiencing GERD are lifestyle modifications (adjustments to feeding and positioning), medication therapy, and surgical treatment.[3,12]

Infants with ongoing regurgitation and inadequate weight gain are managed differ-ently than infants with basic GER.[3] Inadequate weight gain is a warning signal that additional measures need to be taken and best practice guidelines followed such as the NASPGHAN and ESPGHAN clinical pathway (**Fig. 2**). A history and physical exam-ination are conducted by the health care provider including a 24-hour dietary history noting the amount of intake from formula or breastmilk, the number of episodes, breastfeeding routines, and amount of regurgitation, feeding and formula preparation practices.[3] The health care provider may deal with any issues found during the history

---

Box 3
Case study. 4-month-old infant with GER

Sam is a 4-month-old male infant who was brought by his mother to the clinic for a well-baby check with his health care provider. The mother appeared anxious and stated, "Sam spits up after every feeding. I don't think he is getting enough to drink." He weighs 10 pounds this visit and is 25 inches in length.

1. What additional assessment data should the health care provider obtain during this visit?

2. What is the next step for treating this infant?

3. What teaching do you anticipate be done?

Box 4
Answers to case study questions

1. What additional assessment data should the health care provider obtain?
   A thorough history and physical examination need to be obtained including a detailed feeding history, observing for any signs of GER or GERD or other warning signs, determine how frequently and how much the infant is spitting up. The health care provider will determine the number of calories that are indicated for the infant according to his current age, weight, and length. Assessment of the skin turgor and anterior fontanel should be done to determine the hydration status. The infant is weighed, and a physical assessment is completed, which shows adequate weight gain, a flat and soft anterior fontanel; lungs are clear bilaterally with active bowel sounds. Bowel patterns and voiding are adequate without problems or concerns. The health care provider discovered that the mother is correctly preparing the infant formula and should continue with the current brand. If Sam is still spitting up at the next visit excessively, consider trial of a noncow protein-based formula and/or thickened feedings.

2. What is the appropriate treatment for this infant?
   Sam's diagnosis is with uncomplicated GER. The health care provider determined that Sam has been eating excessive calories during a 24-hour period for his current weight. Therefore, diet modifications will be initiated including decreasing the amount of formula per feeding. He is eating every 3 hours, which is acceptable. Further testing is not indicated since Sam exhibits no other problems and is typically a happy baby.

3. What teaching do you anticipate being done?
   Anticipatory guidance and reassurance need to be given to the mother. She will need to know how much formula to feed Sam and how often. The provider determines volume based upon infant's age and weight. Therefore, the health care provider should instruct the mother to keep a dietary nutritional log of all feedings including amounts and frequency. In addition, the mother should document in the log all episodes of regurgitation. Warning signs will need to be discussed that should indicate a return visit to the clinic for evaluation. Instruct the mom to position the baby supine for sleeping. Reassure the mother that spitting up without other problems is common with infants. Sam will most likely grow out of it by 1 year of age. Instruct her to keep follow-up appointments and explain that Sam's growth and development will be monitored during well baby checks. Sam does not need medications or other diagnostic studies at this time.

---

and physical examination that explain the inadequate weight gain. During clinic visits, the infant's weight should be measured and documentation of the nutritional intake history reviewed.

If the issue of inadequate weight gain persists although the caloric intake is sufficient, the infant may need further evaluation for failure to thrive.[3] Ongoing assessment and immediate clinical interventions can prevent the infant from becoming critically ill. Dietary modifications are the next step such as feeding protein hydrolysate or amino acid-based formula and thickened feedings, which increase the caloric density for a few weeks.[3]

Infants who respond positively to these measures are monitored closely in the clinic setting and receive parental education during follow-up visits.[3] However, infants should be referred to a pediatric gastroenterologist if problems with inadequate weight gain continue. Occasionally, infants may need to be admitted to the hospital for observation and further evaluation. The pediatric gastroenterologist may prescribe acid suppression medication and/or nasogastric or nasojejunal tube feedings to improve infants' weight.[3]

Usually, enteral feedings are not initiated for infants with poor weight gain and regurgitation unless other measures have been tried and found to be ineffective.[4] These

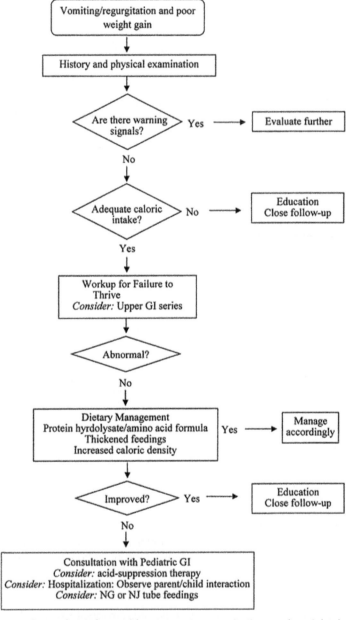

Fig. 2. Approach to the infant with recurrent regurgitation and weight loss. (*From* European Society for Pediatric Gastroenterology, Hepatology, and Nutrition and North American Society for Pediatric Gastroenterology, Hepatology, and Nutrition. Pediatric gastroesophageal reflux clinical practice guidelines: joint recommendations of the North America Society for Pediatric Gastroenterology, Hepatology, and Nutrition (NASPGHAN) and the European Society for Pediatric Gastroenterology, Hepatology, and Nutrition (ESPGHAN). J Pediatr Gastroenterol Nutr 2009;49:520; with permission.)

infants will need to have oral stimulation and allow feedings by mouth if possible while receiving the enteral feedings. It is important to develop a specific nutrition plan for the infant and develop a plan for decreasing and discontinuing the enteral feedings as quickly as possible.[4] Jejunal feedings may be an alternative feeding method to decrease the episodes of recurrent regurgitation or with increased risk of aspiration into the lungs. The infant's weight is monitored to evaluate whether the desired weight is being met and maintained while receiving enteral therapy.[4]

Common medications used for treatment of GERD in infants are antacids and acid suppressants.[3] Studies have shown acid suppressants to be more successful in treatment of GERD, which has led to increased use of proton pump inhibitors (PPIs).[7] Esomeprazole is approved in the United States for use in infants 4 weeks to 1 year of age.[2] It is acceptable to try a PPI or histamine 2 receptor antagonist (H2RA) for a 1 month period of time in infants who cannot communicate their symptoms or those infants with a neurodisability who have regurgitation with feeding difficulties, distraught behavior, or poor growth.[4] After the trial period, evaluate the infant's reaction to the medications and refer the infant to a pediatric specialist for the possibility of endoscopy if the symptoms have not gone away or if the symptoms return after discontinuing the medications. It is acceptable practice to prescribe a PPI or H2RA for infants who are diagnosed with reflux esophagitis by endoscopy. Some medications should not be prescribed as treatment for GERD unless discussed with a pediatric specialist due to possible unfavorable consequences.[4]

Fundoplication is an option for infants with severe GERD who do not respond to appropriate medical management, or if feeding schedules are unfeasible.[4] However, other treatment options should be pursued prior to performing fundoplication (ie, esophageal pH testing or impedance monitoring in addition to esophageal monitoring, and an upper GI series).[4] Yoo and colleagues[5] conducted a study on 11 high-risk infants less than 1-year of age who had Nissen fundoplication surgery because of unsuccessful medical treatment of severe GERD. They found that fundoplication surgery was successful in eliminating the symptoms of GERD in all 11 infants without any problems associated with the surgery. Therefore, Nissen fundoplication is an option for managing GERD when other measures are unsuccessful.[5]

APPARENT LIFE-THREATENING EVENTS

Apparent life-threatening events (ALTEs) occur when an infant's breathing changes quickly and unpredictably by exhibiting periods of apnea; changes in skin tone from pink to a cyanotic, pallor, or ruddy appearance; decreased muscle tone; and/or choking or gagging.[3] Infants with symptoms of acute respiratory complications such as aspiration pneumonitis, apnea, cyanosis, and choking/gagging may have ALTEs, which are often associated with GER. The evidence suggests that GER is rarely the cause of ALTEs. If the health care provider considers GER as a possible cause of ALTEs, then referral to a specialist for evaluation is recommended.[4] Parents need to be educated on use of oral suction to avoid aspiration/aspiration pneumonitis by the infant.

PREMATURE INFANTS IN THE NEONATAL INTENSIVE CARE UNIT

Premature infants are frequently diagnosed with GER during their admission in the neonatal intensive care unit (NICU).[13] Nonpharmacological measures (positioning, thickened feedings, or other feeding options) should be initiated before acid-suppressive medications for treatment of uncomplicated GER with premature infants.[14] Critical care nurses may position infants in prone or on their left side in the hospital setting. However, parents should be instructed to position infants on their backs for sleeping at home to decrease the risk of sudden infant death syndrome (SIDS).[14]

Neonatologists often prescribe acid-suppressive medications such as H2RAs and PPIs for premature infants during and after hospitalization, even though these medications have been associated with undesirable effects such as necrotizing enterocolitis and other infections in the premature infant.[14] It is imperative that the critical care nurse observe for any changes in the condition of the premature infant during assessment or feedings and report any concerns to the health care provider. More research needs to be conducted on the effectiveness and safety of acid-suppressive medications in the premature infant population.[13]

SUMMARY

GER is the most common gastrointestinal problem in infants. Nonpharmacologic management comprises the major interventions for infants up to 18 months of age. Parental education geared at recognizing the signs and symptoms of GER/GERD are essential to maintain a healthy infant. GERD is a more serious condition requiring immediate treatment to prevent respiratory complications, frequent vomiting, fluid and electrolyte imbalances, and failure to gain weight. Infants with GERD need referral to a pediatric specialist immediately for early treatment to prevent further health complications.

REFERENCES

1. Lala SG. Gastro-oesophageal reflux in infants. Prof Nurs Today 2008;12(2):34–8.
2. Czinn S, Blanchard S. Gastroesophageal reflux disease in neonates and infants: when and how to treat. Paediatr Drugs 2013;15:19–27.
3. Vandenplas Y, Rudolph CD, Di Lorenzo C, et al. Pediatric gastsroesophageal reflux clinical practice guidelines: joint recommendations of the North American Society for Pediatric Gastroenterology, Hepatology, and Nutrition (NASPGHAN) and the European Society for Pediatric Gastroenterology, Hepatology, and Nutrition (ESPGHAN). J Pediatr Gastroenterol Nutr 2009;49:498–547.
4. National Institute for Health and Care Excellence. Gastro-oesophageal reflux disease: recognition, diagnosis and management in children and young people. London: NICE; 2015.
5. Yoo BG, Yang HK, Lee YJ, et al. Fundoplication in neonates and infants with primary gastroesophageal reflux. Pediatr Gastroenterol Hepatol Nutr 2014;17(2):93–7.
6. Mitchell A, Lamb K, Sanders R. Gastro-oesophageal reflux in the neonate: clinical complexities and impact on midwifery practice. Br J Midwifery 2015;2(5):323–8.
7. Lightdale JR, Gremse DA. Gastroesophageal reflux: management guidance for the pediatrician. Pediatrics 2013;131(5):e1684–95.
8. Francavilla R, Ciullo C, Cafagno C. The most common errors in the management of gastroesophageal reflux. Ital J Pediatr 2015;41(Suppl 2):A32.
9. Arguin AL, Swartz MK. Gastroesophageal reflux in infants: a primary care perspective. Pediatr Nurs 2004;30(1):45–71.
10. Wenzl TG, Schneider S, Scheele F, et al. Effects of thickened feeding on gastroesophageal reflux in infants: a placebo-controlled crossover study using intraluminal impedance. Pediatrics 2003;111(4):e355–9.

11. Winter HS. Gastroesophageal reflux in infants. In: Update. 2017. Available at: http://www.uptodate.com/contents/gastroesophageal-reflux-in-infants/print?source=sear. Accessed June 28, 2017.

12. Quitadamo P, Miele E, Alongi A, et al. Italian survey on general pediatricians' approach to children with gastroesophageal reflux symptoms. Eur J Pediatr 2015;174:91–6.

13. D'Agostino JA, Passarella M, Martin AE, et al. Use of gastroesophageal reflux medications in premature infants after NICU discharge. Pediatrics 2016;138(6): e20161977.

14. Corvaglia L, Martini S, Aceti A, et al. Nonpharmacological management of gastro-esophageal reflux in preterm infants. Biomed Res Int 2013;2013:141967.

Moving?

Make sure your subscription moves with you!

To notify us of your new address, find your **Clinics Account Number** (located on your mailing label above your name), and contact customer service at:

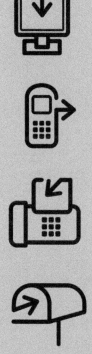

Email: journalscustomerservice-usa@elsevier.com

800-654-2452 (subscribers in the U.S. & Canada)
314-447-8871 (subscribers outside of the U.S. & Canada)

Fax number: 314-447-8029

Elsevier Health Sciences Division
Subscription Customer Service
3251 Riverport Lane
Maryland Heights, MO 63043

*To ensure uninterrupted delivery of your subscription, please notify us at least 4 weeks in advance of move.

Printed and bound by CPI Group (UK) Ltd, Croydon, CR0 4YY

03/10/2024

01040495-0016